# Shopper's Guide to GI Values 2010

## About the authors

**Jennie Brand-Miller, Ph.D.**, one of the world's foremost authorities on carbohydrates and the glycemic index, has championed the GI approach to nutrition for more than 25 years. Professor of Nutrition at the University of Sydney and past president of the Nutrition Society of Australia, in 2004 Brand-Miller was awarded Australia's prestigious ATSE Clunies Ross Award for her commitment to advancing science and technology. She is an in-demand speaker at scientific conferences and her laboratory at the University of Sydney is one of the world's busiest GI-testing centers. Professor Brand-Miller is coauthor of the more than fifteen books in the internationally bestselling *New Glucose Revolution* series, which has more than 3.5 million copies in print worldwide.

**Kaye Foster-Powell, M Nutr & Diet,** an accredited dietitian-nutritionist with extensive experience in diabetes management, is the coauthor, with Dr. Brand-Miller and Fiona Atkinson, of the authoritative tables of GI and glycemic load values published in *Diabetes Care*. Foster-Powell is also coauthor with Brand-Miller of the more than fifteen books in the internationally bestselling *New Glucose Revolution* series.

**Fiona Atkinson** is a research dietitian and the manager of the University of Sydney's Glycemic Index Research Service (SUGiRS). Along with Jennie Brand-Miller and Kaye Foster-Powell, she is the author of the authoritative tables of GI and glycemic load values published in *Diabetes Care*. She is pursuing a Ph.D. at the University of Sydney focusing on the glycemic index.

# Other Titles in the New Glucose Revolution Series

**For the definitive overview of the glycemic index . . .**

**For a focus on recipes, shopping, and the GI in the larger nutrition picture . . .**

**For a basic introduction to the GI plus the top 100 low GI foods . . .**

**For a focus on weight loss . . .**

**For a focus on the GI and specific health conditions . . .**

To stay up to date with the latest research on carbohydrates, the GI, and your health, and the latest books in the series, check out the free online monthly newsletter *GI News*, produced by Dr. Jennie Brand-Miller's GI Group at the University of Sydney: http://ginews.blogspot.com

THE NEW GLUCOSE REVOLUTION

# Shopper's Guide to GI Values 2010

The Authoritative Source
of Glycemic Index Values
for More than 1,300 Foods

**Dr. Jennie Brand-Miller
and Kaye Foster-Powell
with Fiona Atkinson**

Da Capo
LIFE
LONG

A MEMBER OF THE
PERSEUS BOOKS GROUP

This edition is being published in somewhat different form in Australia in 2010 by Hodder Australia, an imprint of Hachette Livre Australia Pty Ltd. This edition is published by arrangement with Hachette Livre Australia Pty Ltd.

The chapter "Sugars and Sweeteners" (pages 79–88) first appeared in *The New Glucose Revolution for Diabetes*. It has been modified for this edition.

Set in 10 point Berkeley by the Perseus Books Group

Cataloging-in-Publication data for this book is available from the Library of Congress.

First Da Capo Press edition 2010
ISBN-13 978-07382-1368-2

Published by Da Capo Press
A Member of the Perseus Books Group
www.dacapopress.com

Note: The information in this book is true and complete to the best of our knowledge. This book is intended only as an informative guide for those wishing to know more about health issues. In no way is this book intended to replace, countermand, or conflict with the advice given to you by your own physician. The ultimate decision concerning care should be made between you and your doctor. We strongly recommend you follow his or her advice. Information in this book is general and is offered with no guarantees on the part of the authors or Da Capo Press. The authors and publisher disclaim all liability in connection with the use of this book. The names and identifying details of people associated with events described in this book have been changed. Any similarity to actual persons is coincidental.

10  9  8  7  6  5  4  3  2  1

# Contents

# Shopper's Guide to GI Values 2010

### 10 steps to a healthy low GI diet for everybody, every day, every meal

- ❏ Eat seven or more servings of fruit and vegetables every day
- ❏ Eat low GI breads and cereals, especially whole-grain versions
- ❏ Eat more legumes including soybeans, chickpeas, and lentils
- ❏ Eat nuts regularly
- ❏ Eat more fish and seafood
- ❏ Eat lean red meat, skinless chicken, and eggs
- ❏ Eat low fat dairy foods or calcium-enriched soy products
- ❏ Eat less saturated fat and replace bad fats with good mono- and polyunsaturated fats
- ❏ Moderate your alcohol intake
- ❏ Minimize your use of salt

# Understanding
# the GI

# Using the Shopper's Guide

We have put together this handy guide full of GI values to help you put those low GI smart carb food choices into your shopping cart and on your plate. By doing so, you'll satisfy your hunger, increase your energy levels, and eliminate your desire to eat more than you should.

Some foods that have been tested by accredited laboratories display the certified GI symbol. But what about the rest? With tables listing the GI of hundreds of foods—from breads and breakfast bars to fruit juice, fruit, and vegetables—this book will save you time in the supermarket by directing you to the best low GI foods available.

You can use the GI tables on pages 96–275 to:

❏ find the GI of your favorite foods

❏ compare foods within a category (two types of bread, for example)

❏ improve your diet by finding a low GI substitute for high GI foods

❏ put together a low GI meal

❏ shop for low GI foods

### The GI explained

The GI is a physiologically based measure of the effect carbohydrates have on blood glucose levels. It provides an easy and delicious way to eat a healthy diet and, at the same time, control fluctuations in blood glucose. After testing hundreds of foods around the world, scientists have now found that foods with a low GI will have less of an effect on blood glucose levels than foods with a high GI.

❑ Carbohydrates that break down rapidly during digestion, releasing glucose quickly into the bloodstream, have a high GI.

❑ Carbohydrates that break down slowly, releasing glucose gradually into the bloodstream, have a low GI.

The rate of carbohydrate digestion has important implications for everybody. For most people, foods with a low GI have advantages over those with a high GI. They can:

❑ Improve blood glucose control

❑ Increase satiety, as they are more filling and satisfying and reduce appetite

❑ Facilitate weight loss

❑ Improve blood fat profiles

❑ Reduce risks of developing diabetes, heart disease, and certain types of cancer

## What are the benefits of a low GI diet?

Knowing the GI values of individual foods is your key to the enormous health benefits of a low GI diet.

Low GI eating has science on its side. It's not a fad diet. There are no strict rules or regimens to follow. It's essentially about making simple adjustments to your usual eating habits—such as swapping one type of bread or breakfast cereal for another.

You'll find that you can live with it for life.

Low GI eating:

❑ Reduces your insulin levels and helps you burn fat
❑ Lowers your cholesterol levels
❑ Helps control your appetite
❑ Halves your risk of heart disease and diabetes
❑ Is suitable for your whole family
❑ Means you are eating foods closer to the way nature intended
❑ Doesn't defy common sense!

Not only that: you will feel better and have more energy— and you don't have to deprive or discipline yourself. A low GI diet is easy and has particular benefits for people who are overweight or have diabetes, hypertension, elevated blood fats, heart disease, or the metabolic syndrome (Syndrome X).

Understanding the GI of foods helps you choose the right amount of carbohydrate and the right sort of carbohydrate for your long-term health and well-being.

A low GI diet has been scientifically proven to help people:

❏ With type 1 diabetes
❏ With type 2 diabetes
❏ With gestational diabetes (diabetes during pregnancy)
❏ Who are overweight
❏ Who have a normal weight but excess abdominal fat (central obesity or a potbelly)
❏ Whose blood glucose levels are higher than desirable
❏ Who have been told they have prediabetes, "impaired glucose tolerance," or a "touch of diabetes"
❏ With high levels of triglycerides and low levels of HDL cholesterol ("good" cholesterol)
❏ With metabolic syndrome (insulin resistance syndrome or Syndrome X)
❏ Who suffer from polycystic ovarian syndrome (PCOS)
❏ Who suffer from fatty liver disease (NAFLD or NASH)

If you would like to know more about the beneficial effects eating low GI foods can have on the above conditions, please refer to our other *New Glucose Revolution* books, a complete list of which is shown at the beginning of this book.

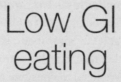

# Low GI
# eating

# Making the change

Eating the low GI way simply involves replacing high GI foods in your diet with low GI foods. This could mean eating muesli at breakfast instead of wheat flakes, low GI bread instead of normal white or whole wheat bread, or a sparkling apple juice in place of a soft drink.

You don't need to count numbers or do any sort of mental arithmetic to make sure you are eating a healthy low GI diet.

## Tips for putting the GI into practice

### The GI only applies to carbohydrate-rich foods

The foods we eat contain three main nutrients: protein, carbohydrate, and fat. Some foods, such as meat, are high in protein, while bread is high in carbohydrate and butter is high in fat. We need to consume a variety of foods (in varying proportions) to provide all three nutrients, but the GI applies only to carbohydrate-rich foods. It is impossible for us to measure a GI value for foods that contain negligible carbohydrate. These foods include meats, fish, chicken, eggs, cheese, nuts, oils, cream, butter, and most vegetables. There are other nutritional aspects that you could consider in choosing these foods: for example, the amount and type of fats they contain.

### The GI is not intended to be used in isolation

The GI of a food does not make it good or bad for us. While you will benefit from eating low GI foods at each meal, this doesn't have to be at the exclusion of all others.

High GI foods like potatoes and bread still make valuable nutritional contributions to our diet. And low GI foods like pastry that are high in saturated fat are no better for us because of their low GI. The nutritional benefits of different foods are many and varied, and it is advisable for you to base your food choices on the overall nutritional content of a food, particularly considering the saturated fat, salt, and fiber in addition to GI.

### You don't need to add up the GI each day

In some of our early books we included sample menus and calculated an estimated GI for the day. As our understanding of the GI grew and we talked to our clients and heard from our readers, we realized this made life complicated for them. No calculations are necessary! Although we can predict the GI of a menu for the whole day, we can't predict the GI of many recipes, especially those using flour. That's why we now prefer simply to categorize foods as low, medium, or high GI in most circumstances. We have also found that many people who substitute low for high GI foods in their everyday meals and snacks reduce the overall GI of their diet, gain better blood glucose control, and lose weight.

### You don't need to be pedantic about GI values

Whether a food's GI is 59 or 61 isn't biologically relevant. Normal day-to-day variation in the human body could obscure the difference in these values. Generally a variation of more than 5 could be considered different.

## This for that—substituting low GI for high GI foods

Simply substituting high GI foods with low GI alternatives will give your overall diet a lower GI and deliver the benefits of low GI eating. Here's how you can put slow carbs to work in your day by cutting back consumption of high GI foods and replacing them with alternatives that are just as tasty.

| If you are currently eating this (high GI) food | Choose this (low GI) alternative instead |
| --- | --- |
| Cookies | A slice of whole-grain bread or toast with jam or fruit spread |
| Breads such as soft white or whole wheat; smooth textured breads, rolls, scones | Dense breads with whole grains, whole-grain and stoneground flour, and sourdough |
| Breakfast cereals—most commercial, processed cereals including corn flakes, Rice Krispies, shredded wheat | Traditional rolled oats, muesli, and the commercial low GI brands listed in the tables. Look for the low GI symbol |
| Cakes and pastries | Raisin toast, fruited-bread, and fruited-buns are healthier baked options; yogurts and low fat mousses also make great snacks or desserts |
| Chips and other packaged snacks such as cheese curls, pretzels, potato sticks | Fresh grapes or cherries; dried fruit and nuts |
| Crackers | Crisp vegetable strips such as carrot, pepper, or celery |
| Doughnuts and croissants | Skim milk cappuccino or smoothie |

| If you are currently eating this (high GI) food | Choose this (low GI) alternative instead |
| --- | --- |
| French fries | Leave them out! Have salad or extra vegetables instead. Corn on the cob or coleslaw are better takeout options |
| Candy | Chocolate is lower GI but high in fat. Healthier options are raisins, dried apricots, and other dried fruits |
| Muesli bars | Try a nut bar or dried fruit and nut mix. Look for the low GI symbol |
| Potatoes | Prepare smaller amounts of potato and add some sweet potato or sweet corn. Canned new potatoes are an easy and lower GI option. You can also try sweet potato, yam, taro, or baby new potatoes—or just replace with other low GI or no-GI vegetables |
| Rice, especially large servings of it in dishes such as risotto, and fried rice | Try Basmati or Converted Long Grain Rice, pearled barley, cracked wheat (bulgur), quinoa, pasta, or noodles |
| Soft drink and fruit juice drink | Use a diet variety if you drink these often. Fruit juice has a lower GI (but it is not a lower calorie option). Water is best |
| Sugar | Moderate the quantity. Consider 100% pure floral honey, apple juice, and fructose as alternatives |

## Your GI Q&A

**Does low carb automatically mean low GI?**

Not at all. Low carb is *just about quantity*; it simply means that a food or meal does not contain much carbohydrate at all. It says nothing about the quality of the carbs in the food or meal on your plate. You could be eating a low carb meal, but the carbs have a medium or high GI. Low GI, on the other hand, is *all about quality*. Whether you are a moderate or high carb eater, low GI carbs (whole-grain breads, legumes/beans, many fruits and vegetables) will have significant health benefits—promoting weight control, reducing your blood glucose and insulin levels throughout the day, and increasing your sense of feeling full and satisfied after eating. We suggest that you make the most of quality carbs and reap the add-on health benefits such as:

❑ Vitamin E from whole-grain cereals

❑ Vitamin C, beta-carotene, and potassium from fruits and vegetables

❑ Vitamin B6 from bananas and whole-grain cereals

❑ Pantothenic acid, zinc, iron, and magnesium from whole grains and legumes

❑ Antioxidants and phytochemicals from all plant foods

❑ Fiber, which comes from all of the above and doesn't come from any animal food

**Why do many high-fiber foods have a high GI value?**
Dietary fiber is not one chemical constituent like fat and protein. It is composed of many different sorts of molecules and can be divided into soluble and insoluble types. Soluble fiber is often viscous (thick and jelly-like) in solution and remains viscous even in the small intestine. For this reason it makes it harder for enzymes to move around and digest the food. Foods with more-soluble fiber, like apples, oats, and beans, therefore have low GI values.

Insoluble fiber, on the other hand, is not viscous and doesn't slow digestion unless it's acting like a fence to inhibit access by enzymes (e.g., the bran around intact kernels). When insoluble fiber is finely milled, the enzymes have free reign, allowing rapid digestion. Whole wheat bread and white bread have similar GI values. Brown pasta and brown rice have similar values to their white counterparts.

**Should I avoid all high GI foods?**
There is no need to eat only low GI foods. While you will benefit from eating low GI foods at each meal, this doesn't have to be to the exclusion of all others. When eaten with protein foods or low GI foods, the overall GI value of the meal will be about medium.

## What GI number should a person aim for when trying to diet?

The simple answer is there's no formula. You don't need to add up the GI each day. In fact there's no counting at all as there is with calories. The basic technique for eating the low GI way is simply switching the high GI carbs in your diet with low GI foods. So, what you need to aim for is identifying the high GI carbs in your current diet and swapping them for some quality low GI carbs. When you're looking at GI values it's best to compare like with like, one bread with another, for example, rather than "bread" with "fruit." This way you'll be comparing foods of similar nutritional value which will help you to make an appropriate swap from the high GI to the low GI version. Try keeping these simple guidelines in mind:

*Every day you need to:*

❏ Eat at least three meals—don't skip meals. Eat snacks, too, if you are hungry.

❏ Eat fruit at least twice—fresh, cooked, dried, juices.

❏ Eat vegetables at least twice—cooked, raw, salads, soups, juices, and snacks.

❏ Eat a cereal at least once—such as bread, breakfast cereal, pasta, noodles, rice, and other grains in a whole-grain or low GI form.

❏ Accumulate 60 minutes of physical activity (including incidental activity and planned exercise).

*Every week you need to:*

❏ Eat beans, peas, and/or lentils—at least twice. This includes baked beans, chickpeas, red kidney beans, butter beans, split peas, and foods made from them such as hummus and dhal.

❏ Eat fish and seafood at least once, preferably three times, each week—fresh, smoked, frozen, or canned.

❏ Eat nuts regularly—just a tiny handful.

## 3 steps to a balanced low GI meal

**1** is for carb
It's an essential, although sometimes forgotten part of a balanced meal. What do you feel like? A grain like rice, barley, or cracked wheat? Pasta, noodles, or bean vermicelli? Or perhaps a high carb vegetable like corn, sweet potato, or legumes? Include at least one low GI carb per meal.

**2** is for protein
Include some protein at each meal. It lowers the glycemic load by replacing *some* of the carbohydrate—not all! It also helps satisfy the appetite.

**3** is for fruit and vegetables
This is the part we often go without. If anything it should have the highest priority in a meal, but a meal based solely on fruit and low carb vegetables won't be sustaining for long. A plain salad sandwich is a recipe for hunger.

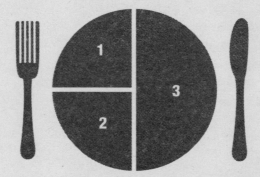

# What's a serving?

*Indulgences*
2 tablespoons cream, sour cream
1 oz chocolate
1 small slice (about 1½ oz) cake
1 small bag (1 oz) potato chips
2 standard alcoholic drinks (a 5-oz glass of wine, 1½ oz
of distilled spirits, or a 12-oz beer)

*Fish, seafood, lean meats, poultry, eggs & alternatives*
3 oz (cooked) boneless meat, fish, or chicken
3 oz canned fish
2 eggs
1½ oz reduced-fat cheese or 1 oz full-fat cheese
3½ oz tofu

*Legumes*
½ cup cooked lentils, chickpeas, beans

*Low fat dairy or alternative*
1 cup milk or soy milk
1 cup yogurt

*Nuts & oils*
2 teaspoons olive or canola oil
1 tablespoon oil-based vinaigrette
½ oz nuts
¼ cup avocado

## Breads, cereals, rice, pasta, noodles, grains
1 slice bread
½ cup cooked rice, pasta, or noodles
½ cup cereal

## Fruit & juices
1 medium piece of fruit
1 cup small fruit pieces
½ cup juice

## Vegetables
½ cup cooked vegetables
1 cup raw or salad vegetables

# Low GI
# shopping

# Planning to shop

The perfect place to get started on healthy low GI eating is the supermarket, whether you are pushing a cart up and down the aisles or shopping online. This is where we make those hurried or impulsive decisions that have a big impact.

Spend a little time each day, or weekly if it suits, planning what to eat when. It makes life simpler. Meal planning is just writing down what you intend to eat for the main meals of the week, then checking your fridge and pantry for ingredients available and noting what you need to purchase.

Our shopping list on pages 24 to 35 will help you stock the pantry and fridge with the staples you require to turn out a meal in minutes. To make your own shopping list, use the same headings. They will take you to the appropriate aisles of the supermarket or to the shops you usually favor. We've included convenience foods such as canned beans, bagged salads, bottled sauces and pastes, canned fruits, and chopped vegetables (fresh and frozen) in the list. There's no need to feel guilty about using these items. Although some convenience items such as frozen vegetables or canned beans may be a little more expensive, the time savings and health benefits can outweigh the costs.

## Making sense of food labeling

Often we're asked questions like: "What should I look for on the label?" and "Can I believe what it says?" There's lots of information on food labels these days, but unfortunately, very few people know how to interpret it correctly. Often the claims on the front of the package don't mean quite what you think.

### Here are some prime examples:

Cholesterol free—Be careful, the food may still be high in fat.

Fat reduced—But is it low fat? Compare fat per 100 grams between products.

No added sugar—Do you realize it could still raise your blood glucose?

Lite—Light in what? It could mean simply light in color.

## Understanding nutrition information

To get the hard facts on the nutritional value of a food, look at the Nutrition Facts table on the package. Here you'll find the details regarding the fat, calories, carbohydrate, fiber, and sodium content of the food.

These are the key points to look for:

**Calories**—This is a measure of how much energy we get from a food. For a healthy diet we need to eat more foods with a low energy density in combination with smaller amounts of high energy dense foods.

To assess the energy density, look at the calories per 100 grams. Solid foods with a low energy density contain less than 120 calories per 100 grams.

**Total Fat**—Seek low saturated fat content, ideally less than 10 percent of the total fat. For example, if the total fat content per serving is 10 grams, you want saturated fat to be less than 1 gram.

**Total carbohydrate**—This is the starch plus any naturally occurring and added sugars in the food. There's no need to look at the sugar figure separately since it's the total carbohydrate that matters most. You might check the total carb if you were monitoring your carbohydrate intake and to calculate the glycemic load of the serving. (See page 49 for more information about the GL.)

**Dietary Fiber**—Most of us don't eat enough fiber, so seek out foods that are high in fiber. A high-fiber food contains more than 3 grams of fiber per serving.

**Sodium**—This is a measure of the unhealthy part of salt in our food. Our bodies need some salt, but most people consume far more than they need. Canned foods in particular tend to be high in sodium. Check the sodium content per 100 grams next time you buy—a low salt food contains less than 120 milligrams of sodium per 100 grams. Many packaged foods and convenience meals are well above this. Aim for less than 450 milligrams per 100 grams with these foods, or at least aim to consume higher sodium types infrequently.

Choose iodized salt because we're all running low on iodine for optimum thyroid function.

Look out for this shopping cart icon for ways to cut your food budget and increase your healthy eating habits.

# YOUR SHOPPING LIST

### The bakery

❑ Fruited bread

❑ Low GI bread

    Whole-grain

    Sourdough

    Soy and Linseed

❑ Muffins, English-style

❑ Pita bread

### The refrigerator case

❑ Cheese

    Cottage cheese / ricotta, reduced fat

    Grated cheese, reduced fat

    Parmesan cheese

    Sliced cheese, reduced fat

❑ Dairy desserts

    Custard, low fat

    Mousse, low fat

❑ Dips

    Hummus

❑ Fruit juice

    Apple juice

    Cranberry juice

Look for fruit juices that are "100% pure" and "unsweetened." And remember not to overdo it—one serving is ½ cup.

Grapefruit juice

Orange juice

❑ Margarine, canola based

❑ Milk

Low fat

Low fat, flavored

Skim

❑ Noodles, fresh

Many Asian noodles, such as "wet" egg noodles, udon, and rice vermicelli, have low to intermediate GI values because of their dense texture, whether they are made from wheat or rice flour.

❑ Pasta, fresh

Ravioli

Tortellini

❑ Soy products

Soy milk, low fat, calcium-enriched

Soy yogurt

Soy frozen dessert

❑ Sushi

❑ Tofu

❑ Yogurt

Low fat natural yogurt provides the most calcium for the fewest calories. Have vanilla or fruit versions as a dessert, or use natural yogurt as a condiment in savory dishes.

Drinkable yogurt, low fat

Fruit or vanilla flavored, low fat

Plain/natural, low fat

## *The freezer*

❑ Frozen berries

Berries can make any dessert special. Using frozen ones means you don't have to wait until berry season.

Blueberries

Raspberries

Strawberries

❑ Frozen fruit desserts or gelato

❑ Frozen vegetables

Frozen vegetables are handy to add to a quick meal.

Beans

Broccoli

Cauliflower

Corn

Mixed vegetables

Peas

Spinach

Stir-fry mix

❑ Frozen yogurt

Frozen yogurt is a fantastic substitute for ice cream. Some products even have a similar creamy texture, but with much less fat.

❑ Ice cream

Vanilla or flavored, reduced or low fat

### Fresh fruit and vegetables

❑ Basics

Carrots

Chili peppers

Corn on the cob

Garlic

Ginger

Lemons or limes

Onions

Sweet potato

Taro

Yam

❑ Fruit, fresh, depending on season

Apples

Apricots

Grapefruit

Grapes

Mango

Oranges

Peaches

Pears

Strawberries

❏ Herbs, fresh, depending on season

Fresh herbs are available in most supermarkets and there really is no substitute for the flavor they impart.

Basil

Chives

Cilantro

Mint

Parsley

❏ Leafy green and other seasonal vegetables

Pile your plate high with leafy greens and eat your way to long-term health.

Asian greens, such as bok choy

Asparagus

Beans

Broccoli

Brussels sprouts

Cabbage

Cauliflower

Eggplant

Fennel

Leeks

Mushrooms

Snow peas

Spinach

Squash

Zucchini

❏ Salad vegetables, depending on season

Arugula

Avocado

Bagged mixed salad greens

Celery

Cucumber

Lettuce

Pepper

Spring onions

Sprouts, such as mung bean, snow pea, alfalfa

Tomato

## *General groceries*

❏ Beverages

Coffee

Flavored milk powders, such as Nesquik

Tea

❏ Breakfast cereals

Low GI packaged breakfast cereal

Natural muesli

Rolled oats, traditional

 Besides their use in oatmeal, oats can be added to cakes, cookies, breads, and desserts.

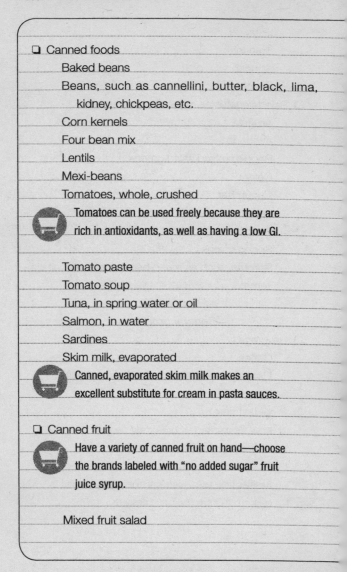

❏ Canned foods

    Baked beans

    Beans, such as cannellini, butter, black, lima, kidney, chickpeas, etc.

    Corn kernels

    Four bean mix

    Lentils

    Mexi-beans

    Tomatoes, whole, crushed

> Tomatoes can be used freely because they are rich in antioxidants, as well as having a low GI.

    Tomato paste

    Tomato soup

    Tuna, in spring water or oil

    Salmon, in water

    Sardines

    Skim milk, evaporated

> Canned, evaporated skim milk makes an excellent substitute for cream in pasta sauces.

❏ Canned fruit

> Have a variety of canned fruit on hand—choose the brands labeled with "no added sugar" fruit juice syrup.

    Mixed fruit salad

Peaches

Pears

❑ Cereals and whole grains

Barley, pearl

One of the oldest cultivated cereals, barley is very
nutritious and high in fiber. Look for products such
as pearl barley to use in soups, stews, and pilafs.

Bulgur/cracked wheat

Use bulgur to make tabbouleh, or add to vegetable
burgers, stuffings, soups, and stews.

Couscous

Couscous can be ready in minutes; serve with
casseroles and braised dishes.

Noodles

Pasta

Pasta is a great source of carbohydrates and B
vitamins.

Rice

Basmati

Converted, long-grain brown or white rice

Quinoa

Quinoa cooks in about 10–15 minutes and has a slightly chewy texture. It can be used as a substitute for rice, couscous, or bulgur wheat. It is very important to rinse the grains thoroughly before cooking.

❏ Condiments

Asian sauces

Hoisin, oyster, soy, and fish sauces are a good range of Asian sauces.

Black pepper

Chili pepper, minced

Curry paste

Dried herbs

Garlic, minced

Ginger, minced

Horseradish cream

Mustard

Pasta sauce

Sea salt

Soy sauce

Spices

Tomato sauce

- ❑ Dried fruit and nuts
  - Apple rings
  - Apricots
  - Natural almonds, walnuts, cashews, unsalted
  - Prunes
  - Raisins
- ❑ Dried legumes
  - Beans

  > Keep a variety of beans in the cupboard including cannellini, black, lima, kidney, soy, pinto.

  - Chickpeas
  - Lentils
  - Split peas
- ❑ Deli items or prepacked jars
  - Anchovies
  - Capers
  - Eggplant
  - Olives
  - Peppers
  - Sundried tomatoes
- ❑ Eggs

  > Buy omega-3-enriched eggs. They are a good way of boosting your omega-3 intake, particularly if you don't eat fish.

❑ Oils and vinegars

Canola or vegetable oil

Cooking spray, canola or olive oil

Olive oil

 Try olive oil for general use; use extra-virgin olive oil for salad dressings, marinades, and dishes that benefit from its flavor.

Vinegar, balsamic and white wine

❑ Spreads

Honey

 Avoid the honey blends, and use 100% "pure floral" honeys, which have a much lower GI.

Jam

 A dollop of good-quality jam on toast contains fewer calories than butter or margarine.

Peanut butter

### *Butcher/meat department*

❑ Bacon

 Bacon is a valuable ingredient in many dishes because of the flavor it offers. You can make a little bacon go a long way by trimming off all fat and chopping it finely. Lean ham is often a more economical and leaner way to go.

- ❏ Beef, lean
- ❏ Chicken
  Skinless chicken breast or drumsticks
- ❏ Fish
  Any type of fresh fish
- ❏ Ground beef, lean
- ❏ Ham, lean
- ❏ Lamb fillets, lean
- ❏ Pork fillets, lean

## Shopping & Storage tips

### Cheese

Any reduced fat cheese is great to keep handy in the fridge. A block of Parmesan is indispensable and will keep for up to a month. Reduced fat cottage and ricotta cheeses have a short life so are best bought as needed. They can be a good alternative to butter or margarine in a sandwich.

### Vegetables and fruit

Vegetables are best fresh, so shop two or three times a week if you can and use them within a few days.

Ethylene gas produced by aging fruit and vegetables leads to their deterioration. You can minimize the effect of ethylene by storing vegetables in the fridge in long life bags, which are available in the produce section of supermarkets, or you can use special cartridges (available in some supermarkets) designed to absorb ethylene. Fruits give off more ethylene than vegetables, but vegetables are more sensitive to its effects, so if you have two crispers, keep fruit in one and vegetables in the other.

### Legumes and beans

Whether you buy them dried or opt for canned convenience, you are choosing one of nature's lowest GI foods. They are high in fiber and packed with nutrients, providing protein, carbohydrate, B vitamins, folate, and minerals. When you add legumes to meals and snacks, you reduce the overall GI of your diet because your body digests them slowly. This is primarily because their starch breaks down relatively slowly (or incompletely) during cooking and they contain tannins and enzyme inhibitors that also slow digestion.

Although they have an excellent shelf life, old beans take longer to cook than young, which is why it's a good idea to buy them from shops where you know turnover is brisk. Once home, store them in airtight containers in a cool, dry place—they will keep their color better.

### Preparing dried legumes

1. **Wash** Wash thoroughly in a colander or sieve first, keeping an eye out for any small stones or "foreign" material (especially with lentils).
2. **Soak** Soaking plumps the beans, makes them softer and tastier, and reduces cooking times a little. Place them in a saucepan, cover with about three times their volume of cold water and soak overnight or for at least four hours. As a rule of thumb, the larger the seed, the longer the soaking time required. There's no need to soak lentils or split peas.
3. **Cook** Drain, rinse thoroughly, then add fresh water—two to three times the volume of the legumes. Bring to a boil then reduce the heat and simmer until tender. Generally, you will need to simmer lentils and peas for 45–60 minutes

and beans and chickpeas for 1–2 hours, but check the recipe instructions. A couple of points to keep in mind:

❏ Adding salt to the water during cooking will slow down water absorption and the legumes will take longer to cook.

❏ Make sure that legumes are tender before you add acidic flavorings such as lemon juice or tomatoes. Once they are in an acid medium they won't get any softer no matter how long you cook them.

Time-saving tips

❏ If you don't have time to soak legumes overnight, add three times the volume of water to rinsed beans, bring to a boil for a few minutes, and then remove from the heat and soak for an hour. Drain, rinse, and add fresh water then cook as usual.

❏ Cooked legumes freeze well. Prepare a large quantity of beans or chickpeas and freeze in small batches to use as required.

❏ Store soaked or cooked beans in an airtight container in the fridge. They will keep for several days.

## Noodles

You can buy noodles fresh, dried, or boiled (wet). Fresh and boiled noodles will be in the refrigerated section in your supermarket or Asian grocery store. Use them as soon as possible after purchase or store in the refrigerator for a day or two. Dried noodles are handy to have in the pantry for quick and easy meals in minutes. They will keep for several months, provided you haven't opened the package. Egg noodles are made from wheat flour and eggs. They are readily available dried, and you can find fresh egg noodles in the refrigerator section of the supermarket or Asian grocery store. "Wet" egg noodles will be in the refrigerated section too. Instant noodles are usually precooked and dehydrated egg noodles. Check the label as they are sometimes fried.

## Spices

Most spices, including ground cumin, turmeric, cinnamon, paprika, and nutmeg, should be bought in small quantities because they lose pungency with age and incorrect storage. Keep them in dark, airtight containers.

## Your shopping Q&A

**How can I feed a big family with cost-effective, no-hassle low GI foods?**

Feeding a big family on a budget can be hard. But low GI eating often means making a move back to the inexpensive, filling, and healthy staple foods that our parents and grandparents enjoyed. This includes traditional oats for oatmeal, legumes such as beans, chickpeas, and lentils (available in cans), cereal grains like barley, and of course plenty of fresh vegetables and fruit, which naturally have a low GI. Some of these foods may take a little more time to prepare than high GI processed, packaged, and pricey "convenience" foods piled high on supermarket shelves, but the savings will be considerable and the health benefits immeasurable. For a list of the top 100 low GI foods, check out *The New Glucose Revolution Guide to Low GI Eating Made Easy*. This book also includes plenty of ideas for using these foods in everyday meals.

**I have recently been diagnosed with celiac disease on top of diabetes. Any suggestions for foods that are both low GI and gluten-free foods?**

This is not as hard as you may think. If you like Asian food—Indian dhals, stir-fries with rice, sushi, noodles—you're in luck, because they are all low GI. Choose vermicelli noodles prepared from rice or mung beans and low GI rices such as basmati. Use sweet potato instead of white potato, use all manner of vegetables without any regard for their GI. Choose fruits and dairy for their low GI. If you can tolerate dairy products, then take advantage of them for their universal low GI. If lactose intolerance is a problem, reach for live cultured yogurts and lactose-hydrolyzed milks. Even ice cream can be enjoyed if you ingest a few drops of lactase enzyme (Lactaid) first.

**I love to bake. If I make my own bread (or dumplings, pancakes, muffins, etc.), which flours, if any, are low GI?**

To date there are no GI ratings for refined flour, whether it's made from wheat, soy, or other grains. This is because the GI rating of a food must be tested physiologically, that is, in real people. So far we haven't had volunteers willing to tuck into 50 gram portions of flour on three occasions! What we do know, however, is that bakery products such as scones, cakes, biscuits, doughnuts, and pastries made from refined flour, whether it's white or whole wheat, are quickly digested and absorbed.

What should you do with your own baking? Try to increase the soluble fiber content by partially substituting flour with oat bran, rice bran, or rolled oats and increase the bulkiness of the product with dried fruit, nuts, muesli, All-Bran, or unprocessed bran. Don't think of it as a challenge. It's an opportunity for some creative cooking. See some of our recipes in *The Low GI Diet Cookbook*, *The New Glucose Low GI Vegetarian Cookbook*, and *The New Glucose Revolution Low GI Family Cookbook*.

## Low GI Breads and Breakfast Cereals

Did you know that the type of bread and cereal you eat affects the overall GI of your diet the most? Why? Well, cereal grains such as rice, wheat, oats, barley, and rye and products made from them such as bread and breakfast cereals are the most concentrated sources of carbohydrate in our diet.

A simple swap is all it takes to reduce the GI of your diet. To get started, replace some of those high GI breads and breakfast cereals with low GI carbs that will trickle fuel into your engine. Here's a list of the low GI breads and breakfast cereals you will find in your local supermarket, or shopping center.

| Breads | GI |
|---|---|
| ⓖ 9 Grain Loaf | 43 |
| Spelt Multigrain | 54 |
| Flaxseed and Soy | 55 |
| Oat Bran and Honey | 45 |
| Sourdough Rye Bread | 48 |
| Sourdough Wheat | 54 |
| **Breakfast cereals and bars** | **GI** |
| All-Bran, Kellogg's | 49 |
| Frosted Flakes | 55 |
| Muesli, natural | 40 |
| Oatmeal, from steel cut oats | 52 |
| Muesli bar, chewy, with chocolate chips, or fruit | 54 |

# How do you know if it's truly low GI?

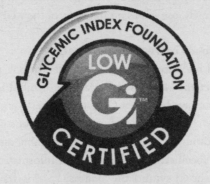

The GI symbol makes healthy shopping easier. This symbol means that the food has been assessed by the experts. It's your guarantee that the GI value stated near the nutrition information table is reliable.

Foods that carry the certified GI symbol have also been judged against a range of nutrient criteria so you can be sure that the food is a healthy nutritional choice for its food group.

In the tables, you'll see that we have highlighted ⓖ the products that carry the GI symbol

## Why put the GI symbol on food labels?

Up until now, people have had to rely on published lists of the glycemic index of foods to help them decide which carbohydrate foods to eat. The GI symbol helps identify foods that provide the GI value. Placing the GI value directly on the label of foods makes it much easier for you to choose foods on the basis of their GI.

## Which foods carry the GI symbol?

Low and medium GI foods carry the symbol, provided they meet the nutrient criteria. The symbol identifies foods that have had their GI tested properly, and that are a healthy choice for their food category. The GI ranking (low/medium) is stated beneath the symbol and the GI value is specified near the nutrition information panel. To carry the GI symbol the food has to be independently tested following a standardized international method.

## Is the GI symbol an indication that foods are healthy?

Foods with the Glycemic Index Tested symbol are healthy in other respects. To earn the certification, foods must be a good source of carbohydrate and meet a host of other nutrient criteria including calories, total and saturated fat, sodium (salt), and, when appropriate, dietary fiber and calcium.

## Are foods with the GI symbol good for people with diabetes?

If you have diabetes you need to consider the quantity of carbohydrate in your serving of food, as well as the GI. Calculating the glycemic load (GL) (grams of carbohydrate × GI ÷100) is one way of combining both factors. (See page 49 for more information on the GL.)

**How can we be sure the information is accurate?**
Foods in the program are required to undergo re-testing for their GI if there is any change in product formulation. All product labels and advertising that use the symbol or mention the program are preapproved by Glycemic Index Limited. Glycemic Index Limited is not responsible, though, for the accuracy and legality of labels and marketing claims of the foods in the program.

**Who is Glycemic Index Limited?**
Glycemic Index Limited is a nonprofit organization established by the University of Sydney, Diabetes Australia, and the Juvenile Diabetes Research Foundation to run the GI Symbol Program. It represents Australia's peak body of glycemic index research and education. Manufacturers pay Glycemic Index Limited a license fee to use the certified GI symbol on their products and the income is channeled back into education and research.

**Why don't all low GI foods have the symbol?**
A food may make a low GI claim on its label, yet not carry the symbol. It may have been tested correctly (check the tables or the online database at www.glycemicindex.com, or contact the food manufacturer to double-check) but the manufacturer may choose not to participate in the GI symbol program. Also, the food might not meet the other nutritional guidelines as it may be high in calories, total or saturated fat, or sodium, or low in fiber or calcium—check the Nutrition Facts panel.

## What about other labels that claim a food is low GI? Can I trust them?

Claims about the GI of foods are currently not regulated. Manufacturers are free to make claims provided they are not false or misleading. They should print the GI value of the food on the food label to help you to verify the claim. A food with a low GI should have a value less than or equal to 55. There are a number of brands that make low GI claims but do not provide a GI value or definition of what low GI means on the label. Unfortunately, you have no way of verifying whether the claim is legitimate. Without verification, it's probably sensible not to trust the claim because you have no idea whether the food was tested following the standardized procedure by an accredited lab.

Sometimes a GI value may be too low to be true. If a manufacturer is promoting a carb-rich processed food with an ultra low GI and does not carry the certified GI symbol, be wary before you buy. Processed foods such as breakfast cereals and breads and bakery products are very unlikely to have a very low GI. In fact, if the GI is less than, say, 50, we suggest that you ask the manufacturer for the name of the lab that tested it and the method that was used.

You may also see products claiming to be "low glycemic" or "diabetic friendly," leaving it open as to whether it's low GI, low GL, or low glycemic response. Be cautious with these claims as the product could actually be low carb (check the nutrition label). Manufacturers making these claims may not be intending to mislead the consumer, they simply may not understand the difference. It's useful to write and ask what they mean and where the food was tested. There are a number of foods that use low GI logos that are similar to the Glycemic Index Tested logo. Some of these cases have been pursued through legal channels.

❏ Consumers in the USA and Canada can contact the Food and Drug Administration's Office of Compliance at the Center for Food Safety and Applied Nutrition (for the USA) and the Canadian Food Inspection Agency (for Canada).

For more information about the Glycemic Index Tested program and the latest list of approved products go to www.gisymbol.com.au.

## How we determine a food's GI value

The GI is a scale from 0 to 100 that captures how the carbohydrates in foods affect blood glucose levels ("glycemia"). It's based on testing real foods in real people. To make an absolutely fair comparison, all foods are tested following an internationally standardized method. The higher the GI, the higher the blood glucose levels after consumption of a standard amount. The GI rating of a food must be tested physiologically and only a few centers around the world currently provide a legitimate testing service.

Testing the GI of a food requires a group of ten subjects and knowledge of the food's carbohydrate content. After an overnight fast, each subject consumes a portion of the test food containing a specified amount of carbohydrate (usually 50 grams, but sometimes 25 or even 15 grams). Fingerprick blood samples are taken at 15- to 30-minute intervals over the next two hours. During this time, blood glucose levels rise and fall back to baseline levels. The full extent of glycemia (rise in blood glucose) is assessed by measuring the area under the curve using a computer algorithm.

There will be some variation between subjects, but if we were to test them again and again, all subjects would tend to move toward the average of the whole group.

## What is the glycemic load?

Your blood glucose rises and falls when you eat a food or meal containing carbohydrate. How high it rises and how long it remains high depends on the quality of the carbohydrate (its glycemic index value or GI) as well as the quantity of carbohydrate in your meal. Researchers at Harvard University came up with a term that combines these two factors—glycemic load (GL).

Some people think that GL should be used instead of GI when comparing foods because it reflects the glycemic impact of both the quantity and quality of carbohydrate in a food. But more often than not, it's low GI, not low GL, that predicts good health outcomes, the reason being that following the low glycemic load (GL) route can lead you straight to a low carb diet: for example, fatty meats and butter have a low GL. But if you eat plenty of low GI foods, you'll find that you are automatically reducing the GL of your diet and, at the same time, you'll feel fuller for longer.

We also emphasize that there's no need to get overly technical about this. Think of the GI as a tool allowing you to choose one food over another in the same food group—the best bread to choose, the best cereal to choose, etc.—and don't get bogged down with figures. A low GI diet is about eating a wide variety of healthy foods that fuel our bodies best—on the whole these are the less processed and more wholesome foods that will provide carbs in a slow release form.

The glycemic load is calculated simply by multiplying the GI value of a food by the amount of carbohydrate per serving and dividing by 100.

Here's how:

$$\text{Glycemic load} = (\text{GI} \times \text{carbohydrate per serving}) \div 100$$

Let's say you wanted to have an apple for a snack. Apples have a GI of 38 and one medium apple contains 15 grams of carbohydrate. So, the glycemic load of your apple snack is $(38 \times 15) \div 100 = 6$.

If you were very hungry and ate two apples, you would be eating 30 grams of carbs and the GL of your snack would be 12. The GI doesn't change, but you are eating more carbs because you are eating two apples.

## Top 10 carbs for kids

1 Apple: Ideal for the lunch box
2 Baked beans: Quick to prepare and handy in the pantry
3 Berry ice cream: Turns fresh fruit into a delicious dessert
4 Bread: A great snack and better than cookies
5 Canned fruits: Portable snack packs are perfect when out and about
6 Corn: Perfect on the cob and a great addition to mixed veggies
7 Milk: Great for kids on the go
8 Noodles: Easy to prepare and a healthy meal with mixed vegetables
9 Oatmeal: A sustaining start to the day—throw in raisins or banana slices
10 Sweet potato: Steamed, mashed, or roasted, a great alternative to the traditional spud

# Eating
out

# Eating out the low GI way

Whether you think it is compatible with healthy eating or not, statistics tell us that at some point you are going to be eating out or buying takeout food. Eating out can really test your resolve as far as healthy eating goes. Like any food choice, however, the more often we eat out, the more important it is that we choose healthy options. If you only eat out once a month you needn't be too fussy, but if it's three to four times a week, good choices are critical.

## Finding the low GI choice on the menu

### Indian food

The traditional accompaniment for Indian dishes is steamed basmati rice, which is a classic low GI choice. Lentil dhal offers another low GI accompaniment, but make sure they don't add the oil topping (tadka).

Unleavened breads such as chapati or roti may have a lower GI than normal bread, but they will boost the carbohydrate content of the meal and increase the GL.

Our suggestions:

❏ Tikka (dry roasted) or tandoori (marinated in spices and yogurt) chicken

❏ Basmati rice

❏ Cucumber raita

❏ Spicy spinach (saag)

## *Japanese food*

Sushi has a low GI, and any refrigerated rice has a lower GI than when it is freshly cooked. The vinegar used in preparation of sushi helps keep the GI low (acidity helps slow stomach emptying), and so do the viscous fibers in the seaweed. Typical ingredients and flavors to enjoy are shoyu (Japanese soy sauce), mirin (rice wine), wasabi (a strong horseradish), miso (soybean paste), pickled ginger (oshinko), sesame seeds, and sesame oil. Go easy on deep-fried dishes such as tempura.

Japanese restaurants are great places to stock up on omega-3 fats, as dishes such as sushi and sashimi made with salmon and tuna contain high amounts of beneficial polyunsaturated fatty acids.

Our suggestions:

❑ Miso soup

❑ Sushi

❑ Teppanyaki (steak, seafood, and vegetables)

❑ Yakitori (skewered chicken and onions in teriyaki sauce)

❑ Sashimi (thinly sliced raw fish or beef)

❑ Shabu-shabu (thin slices of beef quickly cooked with mushrooms, cabbage, and other vegetables)

❑ Side orders such as seaweed salad, wasabi, soy sauce, and pickled ginger

## Thai food

Thai food is generally sweet and spicy and contains aromatic ingredients such as basil, lemongrass, and galangal. Spicy Thai salads, which usually contain seafood, chicken, or meat, are a delicious light meal. For starters, avoid the deep-fried items such as spring rolls.

One downside to Thai cuisine is the coconut milk, which really raises the saturated fat content of Thai curry. So don't feel you have to consume all of the sauce or soup. The traditional accompaniment to Thai food is plain, steamed Jasmine rice, but this is very high GI so you are better off if you can reduce the quantity. Noodles are always on the menu as well, but avoid fried versions. Boiled rice noodles may be an option. Limit yourself to a small helping or, if you are having takeout, you could cook up some long grain rice at home as an accompaniment.

Our suggestions:

❏ Tom yum—hot and sour soup

❏ Thai beef or chicken salad

❏ Wok-tossed meats or seafood

❏ Stir-fried mixed vegetables

❏ Small serving of steamed noodles or rice

❏ Fresh spring rolls (not fried)

## Italian food

The big plus with Italian restaurants is the supply of low GI pasta with an array of sauces. Good choices are arrabiata, puttanesca, marinara sauces (without cream). Despite what you may think, most Italians don't sit down to huge bowls of pasta, so don't be afraid to leave some on your plate (or order an appetizer size)—the GI may be low but a large serving of pasta will have a high GL. Other good choices include minestrone and vegetable dishes, lean veal, and grilled seafood. Steer clear of crumbed and deep-fried seafood.

Our suggestions:

❑ Minestrone

❑ Veal scallops in tomato-based sauce

❑ Prosciutto (paper-thin slices of smoky ham) wrapped around melon

❑ Barbecued or grilled seafood such as calamari or octopus

❑ Roasted or grilled fillet of beef, lamb loin, or poultry

❑ Green garden salad with olive oil and balsamic vinegar

❑ Sorbet, gelato, or simply a fresh fruit platter

❑ Appetizer-size pasta with seafood and tomato or stock-based sauce

## Greek and Middle Eastern food

In Mediterranean cuisine, olive oil, lemon, garlic, onions, and other vegetables abound. Many dishes are char-grilled and specialities such as barbecued octopus or grilled sardines are excellent choices. You will find regular bread replaced with flat bread or Turkish bread, while potatoes are replaced with healthier options such as bulgur (in tabbouleh) and couscous. Among the small appetizing mezze dishes, you could pick and choose what you like. Many of the choices are healthy, such as hummus, baba ghanoush, olives, tzatziki, and grape leaves.

Our suggestions:

❑ Mezze platter with Lebanese bread

❑ Souvlaki (grilled skewers of meat with vegetables)

❑ Kofta (balls of minced lamb with bulgur wheat)

❑ Greek salad of fresh lettuce, tomato, olives, feta, and peppers, with balsamic dressing or oil and lemon

❑ Fresh fruit platter

❑ Falafel with tabbouleh and hummus with a flat bread

## Tips for those who routinely eat at restaurants

1 *Walk* to the restaurant if possible.
2 Order water as soon as you arrive.
3 Send the bread basket away (unless it's *exceptional*).
4 Order green salad, raw oysters, or soup for an appetizer.
5 Order an appetizer for your main course (or specify appetizer size).
6 Alternatively, eat *only half* of everything on your plate.
7 Tell the waiter to hold the French fries.
8 Share dessert with a dining companion.
9 Drink no more than one to three glasses of alcohol.
10 Walk back to the office or climb the stairs.

### Fast-food outlets

Burgers and French fries are a bad idea—quickly eaten, high in saturated fat, and rapidly absorbed high GI carbs that fill you with calories that don't last long. Some fast-food chains are introducing healthier choices, but read the fine print. Look out for lean protein, low GI carbs, good fats, and lots of vegetables.

Our suggestions:

❑ Marinated and barbecued chicken, rather than fried

❑ Salads such as coleslaw or garden salad; eat the salad first

❑ Corn on the cob as a healthy side order

❑ Individual menu items rather than meal deals—never upsize

### Lunch bars

Steer clear of places displaying lots of deep-fried fare and head toward fresh food bars offering fruit and vegetables. Tubs of garden or Greek salad topped with fruit and yogurt make a healthy, low GI choice.

With sandwiches and melts, choose the fillings carefully. Including cheese can make the fat exceed 20 grams per sandwich (that's as much as French fries!). Make sure you include some vegetables or salad in or alongside the sandwich.

Our suggestions:

- ❏ Dense grain bread rather than white
- ❏ Salad fillings for sandwiches, or as a side order instead of fries
- ❏ Pasta dishes with both vegetables and meat
- ❏ Lebanese kebabs with tabbouleh and hummus
- ❏ Grilled fish rather than fried
- ❏ Vegetarian pizza
- ❏ Gourmet wraps

## *Cafés*

Whether it's a quick snack or a main meal, catching up with a friend for coffee doesn't have to tip your diet off balance. Pass on breads, but if you really must, something like a dense Italian bread is better than a garlic or herb bread.

Whatever you order, specify: "no French fries—extra salad instead" so temptation does not confront you. If you want something sweet try a skim iced cappuccino or a single little cookie or a small piece of sponge cake.

Our suggestions:

- ❏ Skim milk coffee rather than full cream milk
- ❏ Sourdough or whole-grain bread instead of white or whole wheat
- ❏ Bruschetta with tomatoes, onions, olive oil, and basil on a dense Italian bread rather than buttery herb or garlic bread

❑ Salad as a main or side order, with the dressing served separately so you control the amount

❑ Grilled steak or chicken breast rather than fried or battered

❑ Vegetable-topped pizza—such as pepper, onion, mushroom, artichoke, eggplant

❑ Lean meat pizza—such as ham, fresh seafood, or sliced chicken breast

❑ Pasta with sauces such as marinara; meat sauce; puttanesca; arrabiata (tomato with olives, roasted pepper, and chili); and piccolo (eggplant, roasted pepper, and artichoke)

❑ Seafood such as marinated calamari, grilled with chili and lemon, or steamed mussels with a tomato sauce

❑ Water or freshly squeezed fruit and vegetable juices rather than soft drinks

### Asian meals

Asian meals, including Chinese, Thai, Indian, and Japanese, offer a great variety of foods, making it possible to select a healthy meal with some careful choices.

Keeping in line with the 1, 2, 3 steps to a balanced meal (see page 16), seek out a low GI carb such as basmati rice, dhal, sushi, or noodles. Chinese and Thai rice will traditionally be jasmine, and, although high GI, a small serving of steamed rice is better for you than fried rice or noodles.

Next add some protein—marinated tofu (bean curd), stir-fried seafood, Tandoori chicken, fish tikka, or a braised dish with vegetables. Be cautious with pork and duck, for which fattier cuts are often used; and avoid Thai curries and dishes made with coconut milk because it's high in saturated fat.

And don't forget, the third dish to order is stir-fried vegetables!

Our suggestions:

❏ Steamed dumplings or fresh spring rolls rather than fried entrees

❏ Clear soups to fill you up, rather than high fat coconut-based soups

❏ Noodles in soups rather than fried in dishes such as pad Thai

❏ Noodle and vegetable stir-fries—if you ask for extra vegetables you may find that the one dish feeds two

❏ Seafood braised in a sauce with vegetables

❏ Tofu, chicken, beef, lamb, or pork fillet braised with nuts, vegetables, black bean, or other sauces

❏ Salads such as Thai salads

❏ Smaller servings of rice

❏ Vegetable dishes such as stir-fried vegetables, vegetable curry, dhal, channa (a delicious chickpea curry), and side orders such as pickles, cucumber and yogurt, tomato and onion

❏ Japanese dishes such as sushi, teriyaki, sashimi, salmon steak or tuna, teppanyaki (which is grilled) in preference to tempura, which is deep-fried

## Airlines and airports

Airports are notoriously bad places to eat. Fast-food chains, a limited range, premade sandwiches, sad-looking cakes, a lack of fresh fruit and vegetables, and it's all expensive!

In airline lounges you will do better, although, again, the range is limited. Fresh fruit is always on offer and usually some sort of vegetables, either as salad or soup. The bread is usually the super-high GI white French type and with crackers as the only other option, you would do better to rely on fruit, fruit juices, yogurt, or a skim milk coffee for your carbs.

In-flight, unless you have the privilege of a sky chef, meals are fairly standard fare, including a salad and fruit if you're lucky. Many airlines offer special diets with advance bookings and although there's no guarantee it meets your nutritional criteria, it may give you healthier choices compared to what everyone else is having.

Travelling domestic economy these days, it's probably best to eat before you leave, take your own snacks with you and decline the in-flight snack (you really will be better off without that mini chocolate bar, cookie, cake, or muffin, which on some airlines you have to pay for).

Our suggestions:

❏ Fresh fruit, soup, and salad items in airline lounges rather than white bread, cheese, cakes, and salami

❏ Small meals in-flight, rather than eating everything put in front of you

❏ Water to drink, wherever you are

❏ Dried fruit, nut bars, bananas, or apples that you have taken along yourself

# Gluten-free eating out

Eating out on a gluten-free diet can be difficult, particularly as there is often gluten in items such as sauces, stock, dressings, and gravy. It is important that the restaurant understands your need for a meal that is completely free of gluten and it may be a good idea to call beforehand to ensure that they can accommodate your needs.

You may have a local celiac society, which should be able to give you a list of recommended restaurants at which to eat, where you can be confident that they are able to provide you with a gluten-free meal. These are good places to start. Otherwise you need to ask plenty of questions and remember that, if you are in doubt, you are best to leave it out!

Following are some tips to making low GI gluten-free meal choices when eating out.

- ❑ Plain grilled steak, chicken, or fish with a corn on the cob, and salad or steamed vegetables

- ❑ Indian dahl with basmati rice

- ❑ Mexican tacos (if made with 100 percent corn tortillas) with beans, salad, avocado, salsa, and grated cheese

- ❑ Sushi filled with raw fish or avocado and cucumber (no soy sauce)

- ❑ Vietnamese rice paper rolls (but hold the dipping sauce unless you can check if it is gluten-free)

- ❑ Asian rice noodles stir-fried with vegetables, tofu, or shrimp, peanuts, cilantro and lemon or lime juice (check the sauces)

- ❑ Mixed-bean, chickpea, or lentil salads (leave the dressing unless you can check it is gluten-free)

- ❑ Falafel (check they are gluten-free) with hummus and salad

## Your eating out Q&A

### What's the GI of a latte and cappuccino?

Most milky drinks will have a low GI and won't add too many calories either so long as you don't sweeten them with more than a teaspoon or so of sugar and say no to those flavored syrups lined up on the counter. In fact, a latte, cappuccino, or café au lait can be the perfect mid-morning snack and an easy way to help you get your two to three servings of dairy foods a day. Regular or skim milk has a low GI—a combination of the moderate glycemic effect of its sugar (lactose) plus milk protein, which forms a soft curd in the stomach and slows down stomach emptying. Regular full fat milk is high in saturated fat, but these days there's a wide range of reduced fat milks including low fat and skim types. If you prefer soy milk make sure you opt for calcium fortified and reduced fat. Note that rice milk is not a suitable substitute; it has a high GI.

How much milk are you getting with your coffee? Well, to some extent it depends on the cafe and where you buy it. But here are some standard definitions.

❏ A caffe latte is a single shot of espresso with steamed milk—approximately a 3:1 ratio of milk to coffee.

❏ A café au lait is similar except it is generally made with brewed coffee instead of espresso in a ratio of 1:1 milk to coffee.

❏ Cappuccino is traditionally equal parts espresso, steamed milk, and frothed milk.

**How can I stick to low GI foods at parties, work events, or during the holiday season?**
For the right fuel, fitness, and stamina to make it through the nonstop demands of social occasions and the festive season, try these seven energy-boosting tips.

## 1. Make breakfast a priority

To nourish your body and sustain you through the morning, fire up your engine with low GI carbs. A good breakfast recharges your brain, speeds up your metabolism after an overnight fast, and reduces those feelings of stress.

## 2. Don't skip meals

Take a break to refuel at lunchtime to maintain energy levels right through the afternoon. Hold back on the high GI carbs to minimize that post-lunch energy dip. And take time over one main meal every day to make sure you aren't missing out on the vegetables you need.

## 3. Build your meals around low GI carbs

Food is the fuel needed to keep your body and brain energized. For daylong energy, fuel your body with low GI carbs that trickle glucose into your bloodstream. Use the 1, 2, 3 guide on page 16.

## 4. Try to be moderate

Pace yourself on the social merry-go-round by eating and drinking in moderation. If you are planning a big night out, don't starve yourself beforehand. All that does is reduce your metabolic rate. Have a light breakfast and lunch, and before you head off to the party eat a quick and easy low GI snack such as a sandwich made with grainy bread and a glass of semi-skimmed milk or a cup of yogurt and a dollop of fruit.

### 5. Be discerning with drinks

Make water your first choice. Ask for some routinely; chances are you'll drink it if it's in front of you. Go easy on the sugary drinks (they tend to bypass satiety mechanisms) and drink no more than one to three glasses of alcohol.

### 6. Move it

Cut holiday stress in its tracks. Exercise helps to relieve stress (it releases the "feel good" chemicals that negate energy and stress) and keeps your body strong. Get on your bike or into your sneakers and get that heart rate pumping for at least 20 minutes a day.

### 7. Get enough sleep

Get seven or eight hours sleep, so plan for as many early nights as you can.

# Low GI
# gluten-free eating

There is much more to a gluten-free lifestyle than focusing on foods you need to avoid. Eating well is the key to good health for everyone and eating the right foods gives your body the fuel it needs to perform at its best and the energy to get through the day. It's also an important part of managing and preventing other long-term health problems, including diabetes, heart disease, cancer, and a range of digestive problems.

If you have celiac disease and need to follow a strict gluten-free diet, we suggest that you join your state celiac society and take advantage of the up-to-date and comprehensive information they provide for their members on shopping, cooking, and eating gluten-free.

While it is great to see an increasing range of ready-made gluten-free foods making life easier for those with celiac disease, unfortunately many of them are highly processed and some are high in fat and added sugar—two ingredients that are naturally gluten-free!

## What is gluten?

Gluten is the protein found in the grains wheat, rye, barley, and triticale. Oats are frequently grown, harvested, milled, and processed alongside gluten-containing grains, so they may be contaminated with gluten. They also contain a gluten-like protein which some people with celiac disease react to. So, while research is ongoing, oats are currently not recommended for people with celiac disease.

Gluten-free diets also tend to have a high glycemic index (GI). This is because many low GI staples such as whole wheat kernel breads, pasta, barley, and oats are eliminated because they contain gluten. The gluten-free alternatives, due to their ingredients and processing methods, are often quickly digested and absorbed, raising blood glucose and insulin levels and leaving you feeling hungry and often low on energy a few hours after eating. What this means in practice is that many people following a gluten-free diet are rarely satisfied after meals and may feel hungry between meals, which can lead to overeating and weight gain.

In addition, adults and children on a gluten-free diet can miss out on the numerous health benefits of:

❏ Getting enough fiber
❏ Managing blood glucose levels with low GI foods. (See the benefits of a low GI diet on page 4.)

Even on a wheat-free or gluten-free diet, you'll find that there are many low GI gluten-free foods you can enjoy in four of the five food groups:

❏ Virtually all fruits and vegetables
❏ Some whole kernel grains in the breads and cereals group
❏ Legumes of all types in the meat and alternatives group
❏ Milk and yogurt among the dairy foods

There are a number of gluten-free breads, breakfast cereals, snack foods, and pastas on the market. As not many have been GI tested, here are some guidelines for selecting lower GI options.

*Bread*

Most of the gluten-free breads tested, including rolls and wraps, have been found to have a high GI. (At the time of publication, we found only one low GI bread on the supermarket shelves in North America—Ⓖ Country Life Low GI Gluten Free bread (GI = 40).) But here is a tip: check out the ingredients list and opt for breads that include chickpea- or legume-based flours and psyllium. For example, we know that chapatis made with besan (chickpea flour) have a low GI. If you make your own bread, try adding buckwheat kernels, rice bran, and psyllium husks to lower the GI.

*Breakfast cereals*

Most gluten-free breakfast cereals, including rice, buckwheat, or millet puffs and flakes, have a moderate or high GI because they are refined, not whole-grain, foods. But you can reduce the GI if you serve them with fruit and yogurt and a teaspoon or two of psyllium to boost the fiber. If you like cooked cereal, try quinoa porridge (made from whole quinoa grains) or make your own rice porridge (from a lower GI rice). Add psyllium husks and rice bran, along with fruit and low fat milk or yogurt.

*Noodles and pasta*

There are several low GI, gluten-free options available in both fresh and dried varieties:

❑ Buckwheat noodles

❑ Cellophane noodles, also known as mung bean noodles

❑ Rice noodles, made from ground or pounded rice flour

Most gluten-free pastas based on rice and corn tend to have moderate to high GI values. So opt for pastas made from legumes or soy—although they may be harder to find.

*Whole cereal grains*

Low GI cereal grains for those on a gluten-free diet include buckwheat, quinoa, and some varieties of rice and corn. Currently there are no published values for amaranth, sorghum and teff. Millet has a high GI.

*Rice*

Rice can have a very high GI value or a moderate one, depending on the variety and its amylose content. Instant and quick-cooking rices all tend to have a high GI. So, if you are a big rice eater, opt for the lower GI varieties with a higher amylose content such as basmati rice (GI = 58) or SunRice Doongara CleverRice™ (GI = 54).

Brown rice is an extremely nutritious form of rice and contains several B-group vitamins, minerals, dietary fiber, and protein. The varieties tested to date tend to have a moderate or high GI, so try to combine this nourishing food with low GI ingredients like lentils or beans, or even in combination with wild rice.

Wild rice (GI = 57) is not rice at all, but a type of grass seed. Arborio rice, used mainly in risotto, releases its starch during cooking and has a medium GI.

## Legumes (beans)

Dried or canned legumes, including beans, chickpeas, and lentils, are among nature's lowest GI foods. They are high in fiber and packed with nutrients, providing protein, carbohydrate, B vitamins, folate, and minerals. Check canned varieties for gluten content.

When you add legumes to meals and snacks, you reduce the overall GI of your diet because your body digests them slowly. This is primarily because their starch breaks down relatively slowly (or incompletely) during cooking, and they contain tannins and enzyme inhibitors that also slow digestion. So make the most of beans, chickpeas, lentils, and whole and split dried peas.

## Nuts

Although nuts are high in fat (averaging around 50 percent of their content), that fat is largely unsaturated, so they make a healthy substitute for snacks such as biscuits, cakes, pastries, potato chips, and chocolate. They also contain relatively little carbohydrate, so most do not have a GI value. Peanuts and cashews have very low GI values. Avoid the varieties that are salted and cooked in oil—choose raw and unsalted. Also be aware that dry-roasted nuts may contain gluten.

Chestnuts are quite different from other nuts in that they are low in fat and higher in carbohydrate. Naturally gluten-free, they have recently been found to have a low GI, which makes them a great low GI, high fiber carbohydrate food.

*Low fat dairy foods and calcium-enriched soy products*
Low fat varieties of milk, yogurt, and ice cream, or calcium-enriched soy alternatives, provide you with sustained energy, boosting your calcium intake but not your saturated fat intake. Check the labels of yogurts, ice creams, and soy milks, as some contain wheat-based maltodextrins, which should be avoided.

Cheese is a good source of calcium, but it is a protein food, not a carbohydrate—its lactose is drawn off in the whey during production. This means that GI is not relevant to cheese. Although perfect for sandwich fillings, snacks, and toppings for gratin dishes, remember that cheese can also contribute a fair number of calories. Most cheese is around 30 percent fat, much of it saturated. Ricotta and cottage cheese are good low fat choices.

For more information about celiac disease and gluten intolerance plus more than 80 recipes, check out a new addition to our series of books, The New Glucose Revolution series—*The New Glucose Revolution Low GI Gluten-Free Eating Made Easy: The Essential Guide to the Glycemic Index and Gluten-Free Living.*

See page 286 for more help on gluten-free eating.

# Sugars and Sweeteners

Do you feel guilty every time you enjoy something sweet? Do you think diabetes equals no sugar? Join the club. Many people think that if something tastes good, it must be bad for them. And many people with diabetes, and even their doctors, mistakenly believe that sugar consumption is the most important explanation for high blood glucose readings.

While we now know that's not the case, old habits die hard. Traditionally, people with diabetes have been told to replace all sugar with an artificial sweetener and to drink diet soda. It's enough to make some people with diabetes turn their backs on all dietary advice.

But wanting something sweet is instinctive, and hard to ignore. It is part of our "hardwiring." In our hunter-gatherer past, fruits, berries, and honey were our only source of carbohydrates.

You'll be relieved to know that most diabetes organizations all around the world no longer advise strict avoidance of refined sugar or sugary foods. This is one of the happy spin-offs from research on the GI—recognition that both sugary foods and starchy foods raise your blood glucose.

Furthermore, dozens of studies indicate that moderate amounts of added sugar in diabetic diets (for example, 30–50 grams per day) does not result in either poor control or weight gain. Yes, a soft drink can be a concentrated source of calories, but so can a fruit juice or an alcoholic drink.

But a word of caution: there is increasing evidence that energy in liquid forms (both soft drinks and fruit juices) may sneak past the brain's appetite center. For example, if you give people 100 extra calories as solid jelly beans, they unconsciously compensate by consuming fewer calories over the rest of the day. But if you feed them 100 calories in a soda, fruit juice, beer, or other liquid, they don't reduce their intake much at all. Those extra calories can head straight for the waistline. In a recent study at Harvard University, the children who became overweight over time were the ones who were greater consumers of soft drinks and fruit juices.

You can enjoy refined or "added" sugar in moderation—that's about 6–10 teaspoons (30–50 grams) a day—an amount that most people consume without trying hard. Try to include sweetened foods that provide more than just calories—dairy foods, breakfast cereals, oatmeal with brown sugar, jam on whole-grain toast, etc. Even the World Health Organization says "a moderate intake of sugar-rich foods can provide for a palatable and nutritious diet." So forget the guilt trip and allow yourself the pleasure of sweetness.

## What about alternative sweeteners?

Alternatives to sugar are widely used by people with diabetes to sweeten drinks (tea and coffee) and foods (breakfast cereals); to sweeten recipes (for cakes and desserts); and in low-calorie commercial products (soft drinks, fruit punch, jams, jellies, and yogurts).

They do give you sweetness with fewer calories, and usually with less effect on blood glucose levels, but there are differences between them.

Not all alternative sweeteners are the same—some have just as many calories as sugar, others have no calories at all; some are thousands (yes, thousands) of times sweeter than sugar; others are not very sweet at all. One thing they all have in common, however, is that they are more expensive than sugar.

There are lots of brands of sweeteners on the supermarket shelves, but essentially there are two main types:

❑ Nutritive sweeteners, and

❑ Nonnutritive sweeteners.

## What's the difference?

### Nutritive sweeteners

Nutritive sweeteners are simply those that provide some calories and, as the name suggests, nutrients. Sugar, for example, is a nutritive sweetener, but so are things like sorbitol and maltodextrin. They have differing effects on blood glucose levels.

Old-fashioned table sugar stands up well under scrutiny—it is the second sweetest after fructose, has only a moderate GI, is the best value for money and is the easiest to use in cooking. And because it generally has a lower GI than the refined flour used in baking, it can actually lower the GI of many recipes! Less refined sweeteners like raw sugar, honey, golden syrup and pure

(100%) maple syrup also provide small amounts of calcium, potassium, and magnesium.

The sugar alcohols, such as sorbitol, mannitol, and maltitol, are generally not as sweet as table sugar, provide fewer calories and have less of an impact on blood glucose levels. To overcome their lack of sweetness, food manufacturers usually combine them with nonnutritive sweeteners to help keep the calorie count down and minimize the effect on blood glucose levels. This will be shown in the ingredients list on the food label.

The nutritive sweeteners such as sorbitol, mannitol, xylitol, and maltitol, and maltitol syrup, may have a laxative effect or cause gas or diarrhea if you consume them in large amounts. Foods that contain more than 10 grams per 100 grams of these alternative sweeteners, or more than 25 grams per 100 grams of sorbitol, isomalt, or polydextrose, carry warning statements about the possible laxative effect on their labels. These products can be a particular problem for children and adolescents, because of their smaller body size.

Used in sensible quantities, fructose certainly rivals table sugar as a good all-around sweetener. It stands out from the crowd, being sweeter than sugar, providing the same number of calories, but having only one-third the GI. So you can use less fructose to achieve the same level of sweetness, and as a result, consume fewer calories and experience a much smaller rise in your blood glucose levels. Its main drawback is cost.

If you have read alarmist reports about fructose and

blood fats and/or insulin resistance, remember that this research was on rats and mice fed excessive quantities— more than someone with even the sweetest tooth could tolerate. There is no evidence that fructose has adverse effects in people with diabetes consuming normal quantities e.g., less than 100 grams per day.

### Nonnutritive sweeteners

Nonnutritive sweeteners (such as Equal, Splenda, or saccharin) are all much sweeter than table sugar and essentially have no effect on your blood glucose levels because most are used in such small quantities and are either not absorbed into or metabolized by the body. Because they are only used in minute amounts, the number of calories they provide is insignificant.

### What's best to use for cooking?

The nonnutritive sweeteners that are made of protein molecules often break down when heated at high temperatures for long periods, thus losing their sweetness. For this reason, they are not always ideal for baking. The best nonnutritive sweeteners to cook with are Splenda, and saccharin, and to a lesser extent Equal Spoonful.

### Are they safe?

As a group, nonnutritive sweeteners have been studied more thoroughly than any other type of food additive. Questions about the safety of saccharin were raised when it was first discovered over 125 years ago, and its effect on human health has been monitored ever since. The same is true of more recent sweeteners such as aspartame and sucralose. There is no convincing evidence so far that any of the nonnutritive sweeteners on the market have any negative effects on our health.

While the nonnutritive sweeteners available in North America are considered safe for everyone, some health professionals opt for caution and recommend that pregnant women avoid saccharin and cyclamate. This is because both of them cross the placenta into the growing fetus and can also be found in breast milk.

Also, studies in rats have shown an increased risk of bladder cancer due to saccharin use and kidney disease due to cyclamate use. To put this in perspective, remember that saccharin and cyclamate were both used widely after World War II because there was a worldwide sugar shortage, and we did not see an increase in bladder or kidney cancer over that period. So it seems unlikely that either sweetener is a problem for pregnant women or those who are breastfeeding. However, some women still choose to avoid these two nonnutritive sweeteners.

### What about Stevia?

The leaves of this semitropical herb of the aster family are around 30 times sweeter than table sugar but with no calories. As an herb, they can be used fresh or dried. In the dried form, less than 2½ tablespoons of crushed leaves can replace 1 cup of table sugar, although it's hard to be specific, because its actual sweetness can vary. Stevioside, its extract, is 250–300 times sweeter than sucrose and is currently not approved for use as a food but is a dietary supplement in the United States and Canada (see also What about Herbal Therapies? in chapter 40). Stevia (Stevia rebaudiana), native to the mountains of Brazil and Paraguay, first came to the attention of the Western world in the 1800s, but remained relatively obscure until it was used as an alternative sweetener in England during World War II.

**Phenylketonuria and Aspartame**

Food and beverages in the United States and Canada that contain aspartame must carry a warning for people with phenylketonuria. Phenylketonuria is a rare genetic disease, which is characterized by an inability of the body to utilize the essential amino acid, phenylalanine. About 1 in 10,000 newborn babies is affected with the condition. Managing this disease includes sticking to a low-protein diet, with particular emphasis on avoiding foods high in phenylalanine. As aspartame contains a significant amount of phenylalanine, it is not recommended for people with phenylketonuria.

## Blends: the best of both worlds?

Splenda Sugar Blend for Baking is a blend of ordinary table sugar and sucralose, a nonnutritive sweetener. By adding sucralose to sugar, you get the best of both worlds: an intense sweetener with fewer calories, but the cooking properties of sugar. Its only downside is its cost—nearly three times that of table sugar.

# What Should You Do?

Replacing table sugar with alternative sweeteners may have some health benefits but these come at a cost. To achieve the best of both worlds we suggest that you use your favorite alternative sweetener in those dishes that normally require a significant amount of added sugar (half a cup or more). For the rest of the time, just have a teaspoon or two of sugar and enjoy it.

See pages 254–261 for more detailed information on nutritive and nonnutritive sweeteners.

# GI values

# Using the tables

These tables will help you put those low GI food choices into your shopping cart and onto your plate. Each entry lists an individual food and its GI value along with nutritional information for each food—fat (g), saturated fat (g), fiber (g), and sodium (mg). We also list the nominal serving size, the amount of carbohydrate per serving, and whether the food's GI is low, medium, or high.

**A low GI value is 55 or less**
**A medium/moderate GI value is 56 to 69 inclusive**
**A high GI value is 70 or more**

You can use the tables to:

❏ find the GI of your favorite foods

❏ compare carb-rich foods within a category (two types of bread or breakfast cereal for example)

❏ identify the best carbohydrate choices

❏ improve your diet by finding a low GI substitute for high GI foods

❏ put together a low GI meal

❏ find foods with a high GI but low GL

Each individual food appears alphabetically within a food category, like "Bread" or "Fruit." This makes it easy to compare the kinds of foods you eat every day and helps you see which high GI foods you could substitute with low GI versions.

The food categories are listed alphabetically, but if you need to find one quickly, check the category index on page 94. For instance, if you wanted to find the GI value of an apple, then you would look under the food category "Fruit." You could check the page number for "Fruit" in the category index.

The food categories used in the tables are:

❏ **Beans and legumes**—including baked beans, chickpeas, lentils, and split peas

❏ **Beverages**—including fruit and vegetable juices, soft drinks, flavored milk, and sport drinks

❏ **Bread**—including sliced white and whole grain bread, fruit breads, flat breads, and crispbreads

❏ **Breakfast cereals**—including processed cereals, muesli, oats, and oatmeal

❏ **Cakes and muffins**—including other baked goods

❏ **Cereal grains**—including bulgur and barley

❏ **Cookies and crackers**

❏ **Dairy products**—including cheese, milk, yogurt, ice creams, and dairy desserts

❏ **Fruit**—including fresh, canned, and dried fruit (see *Beverages* for fruit juices)

❑ **Gluten-free products**

❑ **Meals, prepared/convenience**

❑ **Meat, seafood, eggs and protein**

❑ **Nutritional supplements**

❑ **Nuts and seeds**

❑ **Oils and dressings**

❑ **Pasta and noodles**

❑ **Rice**

❑ **Snack foods**—including chocolate, fruit bars, granola bars, and nuts

❑ **Soups**

❑ **Soy products**—including soy milk and soy yogurt

❑ **Spreads and sweeteners**—including sugars, honey, jam

❑ **Nutritive Sweeteners**

❑ **Nonnutritive Sweeteners**

❑ **Vegetables**—including green vegetables, salad vegetables and root vegetables (see *Beverages* for vegetable juices)

In the tables you will sometimes see these symbols:

★ indicates that a food contains little or no carbohydrate. We have included these foods—like vegetables and protein-rich foods—because so many people ask us for their GI.

ⓖ indicates that a food is part of the GI symbol program. Foods with the GI symbol have had their GI tested properly and are a healthy choice for their food category.

To make a fair comparison, all foods have been tested using an internationally standardized method. Gram for gram of carbohydrates, the higher the GI, the higher the blood glucose levels after consumption. If you can't find the GI value for a food you regularly eat in these tables, check out our website (www. glycemicindex.com). We maintain an international database of published GI values that have been tested by a reliable laboratory (see page 277 for instructions on how to use the database). Alternatively, please write to the manufacturer and encourage them to have the food tested by an accredited laboratory such as Sydney University's Glycemic Index Research Service (SUGiRS). In the meantime, choose a similar food from the tables as a substitute.

The GI values in this book are correct at the time of publication. However, the formulation of commercial foods can change and the GI may change as well. You can rely on foods showing the GI symbol. Although some manufacturers include the GI on the nutritional label, you would need to know that the testing was carried out independently by an accredited laboratory.

# Category index

# BEANS & LEGUMES

| FOOD | SERVING SIZE | HOUSEHOLD MEASURE |
|---|---|---|
| Baked beans, canned in Barbecue sauce, Heinz® | 5 oz | ½ cup |
| Baked beans, canned in Ham sauce, Heinz® | 5 oz | ½ cup |
| Baked beans, canned in Mild Curry sauce, Heinz® | 5 oz | ½ cup |
| Baked beans, canned in Sweet Chili sauce, Heinz® | 5 oz | ½ cup |
| Baked beans, canned in tomato sauce | 5 oz | ½ cup |
| Baked beans, canned in tomato sauce, Heinz® | 5 oz | ½ cup |
| Black beans, boiled | 2¼ oz | ⅓ cup |
| Black-eyed beans, soaked, boiled | 4¼ oz | ⅔ cup |
| Broad beans, frozen, reheated | 3 oz | ½ cup |
| Butter beans, canned, drained | 6 oz | I cup |
| Butter beans, dried, boiled | 5¼ oz | ⅔ cup |
| Butter beans, soaked overnight, boiled 50 minutes | 5¼ oz | ⅔ cup |
| Cannellini beans, canned, drained | 5 oz | ½ cup |
| Chickpeas, canned, drained | 5 oz | ⅔ cup |
| Chickpeas, canned in brine | 4 oz | ⅔ cup |
| Chickpeas, dried, boiled | 3 oz | ½ cup |
| Cranberry beans, canned, drained | 2¼ oz | ⅓ cup |
| Four bean mix, canned, drained | 3½ oz | ½ cup |
| Green beans, cooked, canned | 2¼ oz | ⅓ cup |
| Green beans, dried, boiled | 4 oz | ⅔ cup |

@ part of GI symbol program     ★ little or no carbs

| CALORIES | FAT (g) | SATURATED FAT (g) | CARBO-HYDRATE (g) | FIBER (g) | SODIUM (mg) | GI | LOW MED HIGH |
|---|---|---|---|---|---|---|---|
| 113 | 1 | 0 | 27 | 7 | 572 | 47 | low |
| 141 | 1 | 0 | 25 | 7 | 659 | 53 | low |
| 115 | 1 | 0 | 23 | 7 | 532 | 49 | low |
| 119 | 1 | 0 | 26 | 7 | 549 | 46 | low |
| 116 | 1 | 0 | 15 | 7 | 542 | 48 | low |
| 114 | 1 | 0 | 18 | 6 | 411 | 49 | low |
| 86 | 0 | 0 | 15 | 6 | 1 | 30 | low |
| 125 | 1 | 0 | 17 | 8 | 5 | 42 | low |
| 60 | 0 | 0 | 7 | 3 | 7 | 63 | med |
| 118 | 0 | 0 | 17 | 8 | 711 | 36 | low |
| 120 | 1 | 0 | 17 | 8 | 11 | 31 | low |
| 120 | 1 | 0 | 17 | 8 | 11 | 26 | low |
| 127 | 0 | 0 | 14 | 9 | 213 | 31 | low |
| 166 | 2 | 0 | 25 | 6 | 416 | 38 | low |
| 123 | 2 | 0 | 16 | 5 | 288 | 40 | low |
| 115 | 2 | 0 | 14 | 5 | 9 | 28 | low |
| 92 | 0 | 0 | 17 | 2 | 1 | 41 | low |
| 97 | 0 | 0 | 14 | 6 | 310 | 37 | low |
| 74 | 0 | 0 | 13 | 3 | 291 | 38 | low |
| 126 | 1 | 0 | 15 | 10 | 9 | 33 | low |

# BEANS & LEGUMES

| FOOD | SERVING SIZE | HOUSEHOLD MEASURE |
|------|------|------|
| Kidney beans, dark red, canned, drained | 3½ oz | ½ cup |
| Kidney beans, red, canned, drained | 6½ oz | ¾ cup |
| Kidney beans, red, dried, boiled | 3 oz | ½ cup |
| Kidney beans, red, soaked overnight, boiled 60 mins | 3 oz | ½ cup |
| Lentils, brown, canned, drained | 5¼ oz | 1 cup |
| Lentils, green, canned | 4¾ oz | ⅔ cup |
| Lentils, green, dried, boiled | 4½ oz | ⅔ cup |
| Lentils, red, dried, boiled | 4½ oz | ⅔ cup |
| Lentils, red, split, boiled 25 mins | 4½ oz | ⅔ cup |
| Lima beans, baby, frozen, reheated | 4 oz | ⅔ cup |
| Mung beans, boiled | 5 oz | ⅔ cup |
| Peas, dried, boiled | 6¼ oz | 1 cup |
| Peas, green, frozen, boiled | 5½ oz | 1 cup |
| Pinto beans, canned, drained | 4 oz | ½ cup |
| President's Choice® Blue Menu™ low fat 4-bean salad | 3 oz | ⅓ cup |
| Refried pinto beans, canned, Casa Fiesta™ | 4 oz | ½ cup |
| Romano beans | 5 oz | ½ cup |
| Soy beans, canned, drained | 6 oz | 1 cup |
| Soy beans, dried, boiled | 6 oz | 1 cup |
| Split peas, yellow, boiled 20 mins | 6¼ oz | 1 cup |
| Split peas, yellow, dried, soaked overnight, boiled 55 mins | 6¼ oz | 1 cup |

@ part of GI symbol program    ★ little or no carbs

| CALORIES | FAT (g) | SATURATED FAT (g) | CARBO-HYDRATE (g) | FIBER (g) | SODIUM (mg) | GI | LOW MED HIGH |
|---|---|---|---|---|---|---|---|
| 98 | 1 | 0 | 14 | 6 | 304 | 43 | low |
| 161 | 1 | 0 | 19 | 10 | 495 | 36 | low |
| 119 | 0 | 0 | 13 | 9 | 2 | 28 | low |
| 119 | 0 | 0 | 13 | 9 | 2 | 51 | low |
| 135 | 1 | 0 | 21 | 6 | 350 | 42 | low |
| 87 | 0 | 0 | 13 | 4 | 419 | 48 | low |
| 96 | 1 | 0 | 12 | 5 | 10 | 30 | low |
| 96 | 1 | 0 | 12 | 5 | 10 | 26 | low |
| 96 | 1 | 0 | 12 | 5 | 10 | 21 | low |
| 126 | 1 | 0 | 15 | 10 | 9 | 32 | low |
| 152 | 3 | 1 | 16 | 11 | 17 | 39 | low |
| 118 | 1 | 0 | 13 | 7 | 16 | 22 | low |
| 113 | 1 | 0 | 13 | 9 | 5 | 48 | low |
| 103 | 1 | 0 | 18 | 5 | 353 | 45 | low |
| 70 | 0 | 0 | 9 | 5 | 320 | 13 | low |
| 112 | 1 | 0 | 20 | 3 | 338 | 38 | low |
| 44 | 0 | 0 | 9 | 2 | 354 | 46 | low |
| 169 | 9 | 1 | 5 | 8 | 629 | 14 | low |
| 242 | 13 | 2 | 2 | 12 | 15 | 18 | low |
| 118 | 1 | 0 | 13 | 7 | 16 | 32 | low |
| 118 | 1 | 0 | 13 | 7 | 16 | 25 | low |

# BEVERAGES

| FOOD | SERVING SIZE | HOUSEHOLD MEASURE |
|------|------|------|
| All Sport Body Quencher | 8 fl oz | I cup |
| Apple and blackcurrant juice, no added sugar | 8 fl oz | I cup |
| Apple and Cherry juice, pure | 8 fl oz | I cup |
| Apple and Mango juice, pure | 8 fl oz | I cup |
| Apple and Pineapple juice | 8 fl oz | I cup |
| Apple juice, filtered, pure | 8 fl oz | I cup |
| Apple juice, Granny Smith, unsweetened | 8 fl oz | I cup |
| Apple juice, no added sugar | 8 fl oz | I cup |
| Apple juice with fiber | 8 fl oz | I cup |
| Banana, honey, and malt flavored milk | 8 fl oz | I cup |
| Beer (4.6% alcohol) | 25 fl oz | 2 cans |
| Blackcurrant fruit syrup (reconstituted) | 5 fl oz | ⅔ cup |
| Campbell's, 100% vegetable juice | 6 fl oz | I can |
| Campbell's, tomato juice | 12 fl oz | I bottle |
| Campbell's V8 Splash, tropical blend fruit drink | 8 fl oz | I cup |
| Carrot juice, freshly made | 8 fl oz | I cup |
| Chocolate Daydream™ shake, fructose, Revival Soy® | 8 fl oz | I cup |
| Chocolate Daydream™ shake, sucralose, Revival Soy® | 8 fl oz | I cup |
| Chocolate-flavored milk | 8 fl oz | I cup |
| Chocolate milkshake, commercial | 16 fl oz | I medium beverage |

@ part of GI symbol program     ★ little or no carbs

| CALORIES | FAT (g) | SATURATED FAT (g) | CARBO-HYDRATE (g) | FIBER (g) | SODIUM (mg) | GI | LOW MED HIGH |
|---|---|---|---|---|---|---|---|
| 60 | 0 | 0 | 16 | 0 | 55 | 53 | low |
| 45 | 0 | 0 | 26 | 0 | 24 | 45 | low |
| 138 | 0 | 0 | 33 | 0 | 10 | 43 | low |
| 126 | 0 | 0 | 33 | 2 | 8 | 47 | low |
| 126 | 0 | 0 | 34 | 0 | 2 | 48 | low |
| 130 | 0 | 0 | 30 | | 8 | 44 | low |
| 100 | 0 | 0 | 30 | 0 | 22 | 44 | low |
| 100 | 0 | 0 | 28 | 0 | 11 | 40 | low |
| 120 | 0 | 0 | 28 | 0 | 8 | 37 | low |
| 202 | 9 | 6 | 23 | 0 | 103 | 31 | low |
| 279 | 0 | 0 | 15 | 0 | 53 | 66 | med |
| 82 | 1 | 0 | 14 | 0 | 11 | 52 | low |
| 38 | 0 | 0 | 6 | 2 | 465 | 43 | low |
| 75 | 0 | 0 | 11 | 3 | 1125 | 33 | low |
| 110 | 0 | 0 | 27 | 0 | 50 | 47 | low |
| 71 | 0 | 0 | 14 | 2 | 118 | 43 | low |
| 240 | 3 | 1 | 36 | 2 | 320 | 33 | low |
| 120 | 3 | 1 | 7 | 2 | 320 | 25 | low |
| 210 | 9 | 6 | 24 | 0 | 151 | 37 | low |
| 478 | 14 | 9 | 68 | 0 | 365 | 21 | low |

# BEVERAGES

| FOOD | SERVING SIZE | HOUSEHOLD MEASURE |
|------|------|------|
| Cinch™ Café Latte weight management powder, prepared with skim milk, Shaklee Corporation | 8 fl oz | 2 scoops powder + 1 cup non-fat milk |
| Cinch™ Chocolate weight management powder, prepared with skim milk, Shaklee Corporation | 8 fl oz | 2 scoops powder + 1 cup non-fat milk |
| Cinch™ Vanilla weight management powder, prepared with skim milk, Shaklee Corporation | 8 fl oz | 2 scoops powder + 1 cup non-fat milk |
| Coca-Cola® | 12½ fl oz | 1 can |
| Cocoa with water | 8 fl oz | 1 cup |
| Coffee, black | 8 fl oz | 1 cup |
| Coffee, cappuccino | 8 fl oz | 1 cup |
| Coffee, milk | 8 fl oz | 1 cup |
| Cola, artificially sweetened | 8 fl oz | 1 cup |
| Cordial, orange, reconstituted | 8 fl oz | 1 cup |
| Cordial with water, artificially sweetened | 8 fl oz | 1 cup |
| Cranberry juice cocktail | 8 fl oz | 1 cup |
| Diet Coke® | 8 fl oz | 1 cup |
| Diet dry ginger ale | 8 fl oz | 1 cup |
| Diet ginger beer | 8 fl oz | 1 cup |
| Diet lemonade | 8 fl oz | 1 cup |
| Diet orange fruit drink | 12 fl oz | 1 can |

@ part of GI symbol program     ★ little or no carbs

| CALORIES | FAT (g) | SATURATED FAT (g) | CARBO-HYDRATE (g) | FIBER (g) | SODIUM (mg) | GI | LOW MED HIGH |
|---|---|---|---|---|---|---|---|
| 280 | 3 | 1 | 31 | 6 | 370 | 27 | low |
| 280 | 3 | 1 | 31 | 6 | 370 | 16 | low |
| 270 | 3 | 1 | 29 | 6 | 370 | 22 | low |
| 156 | 0 | 0 | 41 | 0 | 43 | 53 | low |
| 6 | 0 | 0 | 0 | 0 | 13 | ★ | |
| 3 | 0 | 0 | 0 | 0 | 9 | ★ | |
| 55 | 3 | 2 | 4 | 0 | 42 | ★ | |
| 29 | 1 | 1 | 2 | 0 | 26 | ★ | |
| 2 | 0 | 0 | 0 | 0 | 32 | ★ | |
| 75 | 0 | 0 | 18 | 0 | 28 | 66 | med |
| 4 | 0 | 0 | 1 | 0 | 9 | ★ | |
| 134 | 0 | 0 | 34 | 0 | 6 | 52 | low |
| 1 | 0 | 0 | 0 | 0 | 30 | ★ | |
| 3 | 0 | 0 | 0 | 0 | 20 | ★ | |
| 1 | 0 | 0 | 0 | 0 | 48 | ★ | |
| 2 | 0 | 0 | 0 | 0 | 14 | ★ | |
| 11 | 0 | 0 | 3 | 0 | 30 | ★ | |

# BEVERAGES

| FOOD | SERVING SIZE | HOUSEHOLD MEASURE |
|------|--------------|-------------------|
| Fanta® orange lite | 8 fl oz | 1 cup |
| Fanta® orange soft drink | 8 fl oz | 1 cup |
| Fruit punch | 8 fl oz | 1 cup |
| Gatorade® | 8 fl oz | 1 cup |
| Grapefruit juice, unsweetened | 8 fl oz | 1 cup |
| Hot Chocolate mix made with hot water | 6 fl oz | 1 small cup |
| Lemonade | 8 fl oz | 1 cup |
| Lemonade, artificially sweetened | 8 fl oz | 1 cup |
| Lemon squash soft drink | 8 fl oz | 1 cup |
| @ Lo-Gly Acai Blue | 8 fl oz | 1 cup |
| @ Lo-Gly Pomegranate | 8 fl oz | 1 cup |
| @ Lo-Gly Pomegranate Mojito | 8 fl oz | 1 cup |
| @ Lo-Gly Mango Mojito | 8 fl oz | 1 cup |
| Mango smoothie | 8 fl oz | 1 bottle |
| Malted powder in full fat milk | 8 fl oz | 1 cup |
| Malted powder in reduced fat milk | 8 fl oz | 1 cup |
| Malted powder in skim milk | 8 fl oz | 1 cup |
| Mars Active Energy Drink, flavored milk | 8 fl oz | 1 cup |
| Mineral water | 8 fl oz | 1 cup |
| MonaVie E^MV™ | 8 fl oz | 1 cup |
| Nesquik® powder, Chocolate, in 1.5% fat milk | 8 fl oz | 1 cup |

@ part of GI symbol program    ★ little or no carbs

| CALORIES | FAT (g) | SATURATED FAT (g) | CARBO-HYDRATE (g) | FIBER (g) | SODIUM (mg) | GI | LOW MED HIGH |
|---|---|---|---|---|---|---|---|
| 6 | 2 | 0 | 1 | 0 | 26 | ★ | |
| 128 | 2 | 0 | 30 | 0 | 12 | 68 | med |
| 120 | 0 | 0 | 29 | 0 | 25 | 67 | med |
| 63 | 0 | 0 | 15 | 0 | 118 | 78 | high |
| 84 | 0 | 0 | 18 | 0 | 13 | 48 | low |
| 472 | 1 | 1 | 23 | 1 | 150 | 51 | low |
| 104 | 0 | 0 | 28 | 0 | 42 | 54 | low |
| 4 | 0 | 0 | 0 | 0 | 41 | ★ | |
| 128 | 0 | 0 | 32 | 0 | 28 | 58 | med |
| 140 | 0 | 0 | 34 | 0 | 10 | 31 | low |
| 140 | 0 | 0 | 35 | 0 | 5 | 28 | low |
| 120 | 0 | 0 | 31 | 0 | 0 | 32 | low |
| 140 | 0 | 0 | 35 | 0 | 5 | 24 | low |
| 122 | 1 | 0 | 30 | 0 | 28 | 32 | low |
| 278 | 6 | 4 | 30 | 0 | 206 | 33 | low |
| 230 | 3 | 2 | 30 | 1 | 170 | 36 | low |
| 194 | 1 | 1 | 30 | 1 | 190 | 39 | low |
| 220 | 6 | 1 | 3 | 1 | 97 | 46 | low |
| 0 | 0 | 0 | 0 | 0 | 23 | ★ | |
| 170 | 0 | 0 | 40 | 0 | 20 | 52 | low |
| 170 | 2 | 1 | 26 | 0 | 126 | 41 | low |

# BEVERAGES

| FOOD | SERVING SIZE | HOUSEHOLD MEASURE |
|------|--------------|-------------------|
| Nesquik® powder, Strawberry, in 1.5% fat milk | 8 fl oz | I cup |
| Orange juice, unsweetened, fresh | 8 fl oz | I cup |
| Orange juice, unsweetened, from concentrate | 8 fl oz | I cup |
| Pepsi Max | 8 fl oz | I cup |
| Pineapple juice, unsweetened | 8 fl oz | I cup |
| President's Choice® Blue Menu™ Oh Mega j orange juice | 8 fl oz | I cup |
| President's Choice® Blue Menu™ Orange Delight Cocktail with pulp | 8 fl oz | I cup |
| President's Choice® Blue Menu™ Soy Beverage, Chocolate flavored | 8 fl oz | I cup |
| President's Choice® Blue Menu™ Soy Beverage, Original flavored | 8 fl oz | I cup |
| President's Choice® Blue Menu™ Soy Beverage, Vanilla flavored | 8 fl oz | I cup |
| President's Choice® Blue Menu™ Tomato juice, low sodium | 8 fl oz | I cup |
| Prune juice | 8 fl oz | I cup |
| Rice milk, low fat | 8 fl oz | I cup |
| Slim Fast™ French Vanilla ready-to-drink shake | 11 fl oz | I can |
| Smoothie, banana | 8 fl oz | I cup |

@ part of GI symbol program   ★ little or no carbs

| CALORIES | FAT (g) | SATURATED FAT (g) | CARBO-HYDRATE (g) | FIBER (g) | SODIUM (mg) | GI | LOW MED HIGH |
|---|---|---|---|---|---|---|---|
| 170 | 2 | 1 | 26 | 0 | 118 | 35 | low |
| 86 | 0 | 0 | 19 | 1 | 13 | 50 | low |
| 86 | 0 | 0 | 19 | 1 | 13 | 53 | low |
| 1 | 0 | 0 | 0 | 0 | 8 | ★ | |
| 104 | 0 | 0 | 24 | 0 | 2 | 46 | low |
| 130 | 0 | 0 | 30 | 0 | 25 | 48 | low |
| 70 | 0 | 0 | 16 | 0 | 5 | 44 | low |
| 160 | 3 | 1 | 28 | 0 | 140 | 40 | low |
| 160 | 3 | 1 | 9 | 0 | 150 | 15 | low |
| 160 | 3 | 1 | 16 | 0 | 160 | 28 | low |
| 45 | 0 | 0 | 7 | 2 | 310 | 23 | low |
| 144 | 0 | 0 | 36 | 2 | 10 | 43 | low |
| 122 | 2 | 0 | 27 | 0 | 88 | 86 | high |
| 220 | 3 | 1 | 35 | 5 | 220 | 37 | low |
| 215 | 7 | 5 | 26 | 2 | 77 | 30 | low |

# BEVERAGES

| FOOD | SERVING SIZE | HOUSEHOLD MEASURE |
|------|------|------|
| Smoothie, banana and strawberry, V8 Splash® | 8 fl oz | 1 cup |
| Smoothie, fruit | 8 fl oz | 1 cup |
| Smoothie, mango | 8 fl oz | 1 cup |
| Soda water | 8 fl oz | 1 cup |
| Sprite Zero lemonade | 8 fl oz | 1 cup |
| Strawberry-flavored milk | 8 fl oz | 1 cup |
| Tea, black | 8 fl oz | 1 cup |
| Tea, white | 8 fl oz | 1 cup |
| Tomato juice, no added sugar | 8 fl oz | 1 cup |
| Tonic water, artificially sweetened | 8 fl oz | 1 cup |
| Tropical blend fruit drink | 8 fl oz | 1 cup |

@ part of GI symbol program    ★ little or no carbs

| CALORIES | FAT (g) | SATURATED FAT (g) | CARBO-HYDRATE (g) | FIBER (g) | SODIUM (mg) | GI | LOW MED HIGH |
|---|---|---|---|---|---|---|---|
| 90 | 0 | 0 | 20 | 0 | 70 | 44 | low |
| 203 | 7 | 5 | 28 | 2 | 73 | 35 | low |
| 215 | 7 | 5 | 26 | 2 | 77 | 32 | low |
| 0 | 0 | 0 | 0 | 0 | 61 | ★ | |
| 2 | 0 | 0 | 0 | 0 | 30 | ★ | |
| 188 | 8 | 5 | 22 | 0 | 96 | 37 | low |
| 3 | 0 | 0 | 0 | 0 | 7 | ★ | |
| 16 | 1 | 1 | 1 | 0 | 16 | ★ | |
| 57 | 0 | 0 | 11 | 1 | 753 | 38 | low |
| 0 | 0 | 0 | 0 | 0 | 0 | ★ | |
| 294 | 0 | 0 | 20 | 0 | 51 | 47 | low |

# BREAD

| FOOD | SERVING SIZE | HOUSEHOLD MEASURE |
|------|------|------|
| 3 Grain Bread, sprouted grains | 1 oz | 2 slices |
| 9 Grain muffin | 1 oz | 2 muffins |
| 9 Grain, multigrain bread | 1¼ oz | 1 slice |
| 100% whole grain bread | 1 oz | 1 slice |
| Apricot fruit bread | 1½ oz | 1 thick slice |
| Bagel, white | 1 oz | ½ average |
| Baguette, traditional French bread | 2 oz | 2 slices |
| Black rye bread | 1½ oz | 1 slice |
| Bread roll, white | 1 oz | ½ large (4 inch diameter) |
| Bread roll, whole wheat | 1¼ oz | ½ large (4 inch diameter) |
| ⓖ Bürgen® Fruit and Muesli | 1½ oz | 1 slice |
| ⓖ Bürgen® Mixed Grain | 1½ oz | 1 slice |
| ⓖ Bürgen® Oat Bran and Honey bread | 1½ oz | 1 slice |
| ⓖ Bürgen® Rye bread | 1½ oz | 1 slice |
| ⓖ Bürgen® soy and flaxseed bread | 1½ oz | 1 slice |
| ⓖ Bürgen® Wholewheat and Grain | 1½ oz | 1 slice |
| Cape fruit and nut bread | 1½ oz | 1 thick slice |
| Cape seed bread | 3 oz | 2 slices |
| COBS Bread Higher-Fibre Low GI White Block Loaf | 2½ oz | 2 slices |
| COBS Bread Higher-Fibre Low GI White Block Loaf Small | 2 oz | 2 slices |

ⓖ part of GI symbol program    ★ little or no carbs

| CALORIES | FAT (g) | SATURATED FAT (g) | CARBO-HYDRATE (g) | FIBER (g) | SODIUM (mg) | GI | LOW MED HIGH |
|---|---|---|---|---|---|---|---|
| 120 | 2 | 0 | 17 | 3 | 200 | 55 | low |
| 79 | 2 | 0 | 11 | 2 | 86 | 43 | low |
| 69 | 2 | 0 | 13 | 2 | 167 | 43 | low |
| 90 | 2 | 0 | 11 | 4 | 120 | 51 | low |
| 116 | 0 | 0 | 24 | 2 | 124 | 56 | med |
| 85 | 0 | 0 | 16 | 1 | 152 | 72 | high |
| 162 | 1 | 0 | 31 | 1 | 362 | 77 | high |
| 98 | 1 | 0 | 18 | 3 | 252 | 76 | high |
| 97 | 1 | 0 | 17 | 1 | 188 | 71 | high |
| 99 | 1 | 0 | 17 | 2 | 202 | 70 | high |
| 117 | 3 | 0 | 13 | 5 | 85 | 53 | low |
| 92 | 1 | 0 | 15 | 2 | 155 | 52 | low |
| 94 | 2 | 0 | 13 | 4 | 153 | 45 | low |
| 89 | 2 | 0 | 13 | 2 | 150 | 51 | low |
| 98 | 3 | 0 | 12 | 2 | 146 | 36 | low |
| 90 | 1 | 0 | 14 | 2 | 151 | 43 | low |
| 133 | 4 | 0 | 16 | 3 | 109 | 55 | low |
| 260 | 12 | 1 | 25 | 7 | 264 | 48 | low |
| 170 | 0.5 | 0 | 38 | 6 | 390 | 46 | low |
| 140 | 0 | 0 | 30 | 4 | 310 | 46 | low |

# BREAD

| FOOD | SERVING SIZE | HOUSEHOLD MEASURE |
|------|--------------|-------------------|
| COBS Bread Higher-Fibre Low GI White Roll | 2¼ oz | 1 roll |
| Continental fruit loaf | ¾ oz | 1 slice |
| Corn tortilla | 1 oz | 1 tortilla |
| Country grain bread | 2½ oz | 2 slices |
| ⓖ Country Life Country Grain and Organic Rye | 1¾ oz | 1½ slices |
| Country Life gluten-free multigrain bread | 1 oz | 1 slice |
| ⓖ Country Life low GI gluten-free white bread | 1 oz | 1 slice |
| ⓖ Country Life PerforMAX | 2 oz | 1½ slices |
| ⓖ Country Life Rye Hi-soy and flaxseed | 1¾ oz | 1½ slices |
| ⓖ Cripps 9 Grain loaf | 1 oz | 1 slice |
| Croissant, plain | 1 oz | ½ average |
| Crumpet | 1¼ oz | 1 round |
| ⓖ EnerGI white sandwich bread | 1¼ oz | 1 slice |
| Flaxseed and soy bread | 3 oz | 2 slices |
| Fruit and spice loaf | 2 oz | 2 slices |
| Gluten-free buckwheat bread | 1 oz | 1 slice |
| Hamburger bun, white | 1 oz | 1 large (4-inch diameter) |
| Helga's™ Classic Seed Loaf | 1¼ oz | 1 slice |

ⓖ part of GI symbol program  ★ little or no carbs

| CALORIES | FAT (g) | SATURATED FAT (g) | CARBO-HYDRATE (g) | FIBER (g) | SODIUM (mg) | GI | LOW MED HIGH |
|---|---|---|---|---|---|---|---|
| 170 | 0.5 | 0 | 37 | 6 | 370 | 50 | low |
| 65 | 1 | 0 | 12 | 1 | 51 | 47 | low |
| 74 | 1 | 0 | 14 | 2 | 54 | 53 | low |
| 180 | 2 | 0 | 28 | 5 | 377 | 61 | med |
| 123 | 2 | 1 | 15 | 6 | 125 | 48 | low |
| 81 | 2 | 1 | 14 | 0 | 74 | 79 | high |
| 162 | 6 | 1 | 19 | 1 | 183 | 40 | low |
| 137 | 3 | 0 | 17 | 6 | 172 | 38 | low |
| 111 | 2 | 0 | 14 | 5 | 110 | 42 | low |
| 85 | 2 | 0 | 122 | 2 | 153 | 43 | low |
| 140 | 8 | 4 | 13 | 1 | 126 | 67 | med |
| 78 | 0 | 0 | 16 | 1 | 389 | 69 | med |
| 93 | 1 | 0 | 17 | 2 | 162 | 54 | low |
| 230 | 8 | 1 | 26 | 6 | 364 | 55 | low |
| 157 | 2 | 0 | 29 | 2 | 129 | 54 | low |
| 60 | 1 | 0 | 11 | 1 | 194 | 72 | high |
| 97 | 1 | 0 | 18 | 1 | 188 | 61 | med |
| 106 | 2 | 0 | 16 | 2 | 213 | 68 | med |

# BREAD

| FOOD | SERVING SIZE | HOUSEHOLD MEASURE |
|------|---------|-------------------|
| Helga's™ Traditional Whole wheat Bread | 1¼ oz | 1 slice |
| Homemade white bread | 1¼ oz | 1 thin slice |
| Hotdog roll, white | 1½ oz | 1 roll |
| Italian bread | 1¼ oz | 1 slice |
| Kaiser roll, white | 1 oz | ¼ roll |
| Lebanese bread, white | 1 oz | ½ medium (6- or 7-inch diameter) |
| Light rye bread | 1 oz | ¾ slice |
| Melba toast, plain | ½ oz | 1 slice |
| Multigrain sandwich bread | 1 oz | 1 slice |
| Natural Ovens English Muffin™ bread, | 1 oz | 1 slice |
| Natural Ovens Happiness™, cinnamon, raisin, pecan bread | 1 oz | 1 slice |
| Natural Ovens Hunger Filler™, whole grain bread, | 1 oz | 1 slice |
| Organic stoneground whole wheat sourdough bread | 1¼ oz | 1 slice |
| Pita bread, white | 1¼ oz | ½ medium (6- or 7-inch diameter) |
| Pita, white, mini | 1 oz | 1 pita |
| President's Choice® Blue Menu™ 100% Whole Wheat Gigantico Burger Buns | 2¾ oz | 1 bun |

ⓖ part of GI symbol program  ★ little or no carbs

| CALORIES | FAT (g) | SATURATED FAT (g) | CARBO-HYDRATE (g) | FIBER (g) | SODIUM (mg) | GI | LOW MED HIGH |
|---|---|---|---|---|---|---|---|
| 99 | 1 | 0 | 16 | 3 | 209 | 70 | high |
| 87 | 0 | 0 | 18 | 1 | 1 | 70 | high |
| 120 | 2 | 0 | 22 | 1 | 206 | 68 | med |
| 98 | 1 | 0 | 18 | 1 | 204 | 73 | high |
| 77 | 1 | 0 | 15 | 1 | 161 | 73 | high |
| 98 | 1 | 0 | 19 | 1 | 158 | 75 | high |
| 82 | 1 | 0 | 14 | 2 | 176 | 68 | med |
| 59 | 1 | 0 | 11 | 1 | 104 | 70 | high |
| 77 | 1 | 0 | 14 | 1 | 135 | 65 | med |
| 90 | 1 | 0 | 15 | 1 | 115 | 77 | high |
| 90 | 2 | 0 | 12 | 3 | 90 | 63 | med |
| 90 | 2 | 0 | 11 | 4 | 100 | 59 | med |
| 95 | 1 | 0 | 17 | 1 | 218 | 59 | med |
| 98 | 1 | 0 | 17 | 1 | 158 | 63 | med |
| 82 | 0 | 0 | 16 | 1 | 161 | 68 | med |
| 200 | 3 | 1 | 31 | 6 | 440 | 62 | med |

# BREAD

| FOOD | SERVING SIZE | HOUSEHOLD MEASURE |
|------|------|------|
| President's Choice® Blue Menu™ 100% Whole Wheat Gigantico Hot Dog Rolls | 3¼ oz | 1 roll |
| President's Choice® Blue Menu™ Lavash Whole Grain Flatbread | 3 oz | 1 flatbread |
| President's Choice® Blue Menu™ multi-grain flax loaf | 3 oz | 2 slices |
| President's Choice® Blue Menu™ Oatmeal Loaf | 3¼ oz | 1 slice |
| President's Choice® Blue Menu™ tortillas, flax | 2 oz | 1 tortilla |
| President's Choice® Blue Menu™ tortillas, whole wheat | 2 oz | 1 tortilla |
| President's Choice® Blue Menu™ Whole Grain Baguette | 1¾ oz | 1 thick slice (2 inches wide) |
| President's Choice® Blue Menu™ Whole Grain Chipotle Red Pepper Tortilla | 2¼ oz | 1 tortilla |
| President's Choice® Blue Menu™ Whole Grain Cinnamon Raisin Bagel | 2 oz | 1 bagel |
| President's Choice® Blue Menu™ Whole Grain English muffins | 2 oz | 1 muffin |
| President's Choice® Blue Menu™ Whole Grain Jalapeno Corn Tortilla | 2¼ oz | 1 tortilla |
| President's Choice® Blue Menu™ Whole Grain Multi-Grain Flax Bagel | 2 oz | 1 bagel |

@ part of GI symbol program   ★ little or no carbs

| CALORIES | FAT (g) | SATURATED FAT (g) | CARBO-HYDRATE (g) | FIBER (g) | SODIUM (mg) | GI | LOW MED HIGH |
|---|---|---|---|---|---|---|---|
| 230 | 3 | 1 | 36 | 6 | 450 | 62 | med |
| 250 | 2 | 0 | 50 | 4 | 230 | 47 | low |
| 220 | 4 | 1 | 32 | 6 | 260 | 51 | low |
| 200 | 3 | 1 | 43 | 9 | 250 | 63 | med |
| 140 | 5 | 1 | 29 | 3 | 480 | 53 | low |
| 190 | 5 | 1 | 27 | 4 | 470 | 59 | med |
| 130 | 2 | 0 | 21 | 3 | 260 | 73 | high |
| 190 | 4 | 1 | 32 | 4 | 430 | 35 | low |
| 160 | 2 | 0 | 31 | 6 | 180 | 52 | low |
| 140 | 3 | 0 | 20 | 3 | 130 | 51 | low |
| 200 | 5 | 1 | 32 | 4 | 420 | 55 | low |
| 170 | 3 | 1 | 28 | 5 | 200 | 58 | med |

# BREAD

| FOOD | SERVING SIZE | HOUSEHOLD MEASURE |
|------|------|------|
| President's Choice® Blue Menu™ Whole Grain Multi-Grain | 2 oz | 1 muffin |
| President's Choice® Blue Menu™ Whole Grain Oatmeal Bagel | 2 oz | 1 bagel |
| President's Choice® Blue Menu™ whole wheat soy loaf | 3 oz | 2 slices |
| Pumpernickel bread | 1 oz | ⅔ slice |
| Raisin toast | 1 oz | 1 slice |
| Rye bread, whole grain | 1 oz | 1 slice |
| Schinkenbrot, dark rye bread | 1¼ oz | 1 slice |
| Sourdough rye bread | 1¼ oz | 1 slice |
| Sourdough wheat bread | 1 oz | 1 slice |
| Spelt multigrain bread | 1¼ oz | 1 slice |
| Stuffing, bread | 2¾ oz | ½ cup |
| Traditional sourdough bread | 3 oz | 2 slices |
| Tortilla, reduced carbohydrate | 1 oz | 1 tortilla |
| Turkish bread, white | 3 oz | 2 slices |
| @ Vogel's Original Mixed Grain | 1½ oz | 1 slice |
| @ Vogel's Rye with Sunflower | 1½ oz | 1 slice |
| @ Vogel's Seven Seed | 1½ oz | 1 slice |
| @ Vogel's Soy and flaxseed with Oats | 1½ oz | 1 slice |
| Volkornbrot, whole grain rye bread | 1 oz | 1 slice |
| White bread, regular, sliced | 1 oz | 1 slice |

@ part of GI symbol program   ★ little or no carbs

| CALORIES | FAT (g) | SATURATED FAT (g) | CARBO-HYDRATE (g) | FIBER (g) | SODIUM (mg) | GI | LOW MED HIGH |
|---|---|---|---|---|---|---|---|
| 140 | 3 | 0 | 20 | 3 | 130 | 45 | low |
| 160 | 2 | 1 | 30 | 5 | 200 | 63 | med |
| 210 | 3 | 1 | 27 | 7 | 240 | 45 | low |
| 74 | 0 | 0 | 14 | 3 | 226 | 50 | low |
| 90 | 1 | 0 | 17 | 1 | 74 | 63 | med |
| 73 | 1 | 0 | 12 | 2 | 187 | 58 | med |
| 102 | 1 | 0 | 18 | 3 | 217 | 86 | high |
| 96 | 1 | 0 | 18 | 2 | 211 | 48 | low |
| 62 | 1 | 0 | 11 | 1 | 134 | 54 | low |
| 85 | 1 | 0 | 14 | 3 | 188 | 54 | low |
| 152 | 7 | 2 | 17 | 2 | 410 | 74 | high |
| 218 | 1 | 0 | 42 | 2 | 451 | 58 | med |
| 60 | 2 | 0 | 7 | 8 | 49 | 51 | low |
| 197 | 2 | 0 | 40 | 2 | 425 | 87 | high |
| 105 | 2 | 0 | 16 | 3 | 176 | 54 | low |
| 108 | 2 | 0 | 15 | 3 | 172 | 47 | low |
| 110 | 3 | 1 | 12 | 4 | 167 | 50 | low |
| 106 | 3 | 0 | 11 | 4 | 176 | 49 | low |
| 90 | 0 | 0 | 18 | 2 | 200 | 56 | med |
| 69 | 1 | 0 | 13 | 1 | 143 | 71 | high |

# BREAD

| FOOD | SERVING SIZE | HOUSEHOLD MEASURE |
|---|---|---|
| White bread, high fiber, low GI | 1¼ oz | 1 slice |
| White Vienna bread | 1½ oz | 2 slices |
| Whole grain rye bread | 1 oz | 1 slice |
| Whole wheat block loaf | 2½ oz | 2 slices |
| Whole wheat sandwich bread | 1 oz | 1 slice |
| Wholemeal country grain bread | 2½ oz | 2 slices |
| Wonder White® | 1 oz | 1 slice |
| @ Wonder White Low GI sandwich bread | 1 oz | 1 slice |

@ part of GI symbol program   ★ little or no carbs

| CALORIES | FAT (g) | SATURATED FAT (g) | CARBO-HYDRATE (g) | FIBER (g) | SODIUM (mg) | GI | LOW MED HIGH |
|---|---|---|---|---|---|---|---|
| 86 | 1 | 0 | 15 | 4 | 218 | 52 | low |
| 117 | 1 | 0 | 23 | 1 | 250 | 66 | med |
| 83 | 1 | 0 | 15 | 2 | 211 | 58 | med |
| 164 | 2 | 0 | 27 | 1 | 368 | 71 | high |
| 75 | 1 | 0 | 12 | 2 | 135 | 71 | high |
| 178 | 2 | 0 | 28 | 5 | 372 | 53 | low |
| 69 | 1 | 0 | 12 | 1 | 128 | 80 | high |
| 81 | 1 | 0 | 13 | 3 | 151 | 54 | low |

# BREAKFAST CEREALS

| FOOD | SERVING SIZE | HOUSEHOLD MEASURE |
|------|------|------|
| All-Bran™, Kellogg's® | 1 oz | ½ cup |
| All-Bran® Complete Wheat Flakes, Kellogg's® | 1 oz | ⅔ cup |
| All-Bran® Fruit 'n' Oats, Kellogg's® | 1 oz | ⅓ cup |
| All Bran® Bran Buds, Kellogg's® | 1 oz | ⅓ cup |
| Bran Buds with psyllium, Kellogg's® | 1 oz | ⅓ cup |
| Bran Chex™, Nabisco | 1 oz | ¾ cup |
| Bran Flakes, Kellogg's® | ¾ oz | ½ cup |
| @ Bürgen® Fruit and Muesli | 1 oz | ¼ cup |
| @ Bürgen® Rye Muesli | 1 oz | ¼ cup |
| @ Bürgen® Soy-Flax Muesli | 1 oz | ¼ cup |
| Cheerios™, General Mills | 1 oz | 1 cup |
| Coco Pops®, Kellogg's® | 1 oz | 1 cup |
| Corn Bran™, Quaker Oats | 1 oz | ¾ cup |
| Corn Chex™, Nabisco | 1 oz | 1 cup |
| Corn Pops®, Kellogg's® | 1 oz | 1 cup |
| Corn Flakes™, Kellogg's® | 1 oz | 1 cup |
| Cream of Wheat™, Instant | 6 oz | 1 cup |
| Cream of Wheat™ | 6 oz | 1 cup |
| Crispix™, Kellogg's® | 1 oz | 1 cup |
| Crunchy Nut Corn Flakes, Kellogg's® | ¾ oz | ½ cup |
| Froot Loops®, Kellogg's® | ¾ oz | ½ cup |
| Frosted Flakes®, Kellogg's® | ¾ oz | ½ cup |
| Gluten-free muesli | 1½ oz | ½ cup |

@ part of GI symbol program    ★ little or no carbs

| CALORIES | FAT (g) | SATURATED FAT (g) | CARBO-HYDRATE (g) | FIBER (g) | SODIUM (mg) | GI | LOW MED HIGH |
|---|---|---|---|---|---|---|---|
| 80 | 1 | 0 | 23 | 10 | 80 | 49 | low |
| 107 | 1 | 0 | 21 | 4 | 99 | 60 | med |
| 104 | 1 | 0 | 16 | 6 | 57 | 39 | low |
| 70 | 1 | 0 | 24 | 13 | 200 | 58 | med |
| 70 | 1 | 0 | 24 | 13 | 200 | 47 | low |
| 160 | 2 | 0 | 39 | 6 | 310 | 58 | med |
| 72 | 0 | 0 | 14 | 3 | 66 | 74 | high |
| 86 | 2 | 0 | 15 | 2 | 43 | 51 | low |
| 89 | 3 | 0 | 13 | 3 | 38 | 41 | low |
| 92 | 3 | 0 | 13 | 3 | 37 | 51 | low |
| 110 | 2 | 0 | 21 | 2 | 250 | 74 | high |
| 110 | 0 | 0 | 26 | 0 | 112 | 80 | high |
| 90 | 1 | 0 | 24 | 5 | 232 | 75 | high |
| 120 | 1 | 0 | 26 | 1 | 290 | 83 | high |
| 110 | 0 | 0 | 26 | 0 | 112 | 80 | high |
| 100 | 0 | 0 | 24 | 1 | 200 | 86 | high |
| 149 | 1 | 0 | 33 | 1 | 10 | 74 | high |
| 131 | 1 | 0 | 29 | 1 | 8 | 66 | med |
| 110 | 0 | 0 | 25 | 0 | 210 | 87 | high |
| 76 | 1 | 0 | 15 | 1 | 158 | 72 | high |
| 78 | 0 | 0 | 17 | 1 | 94 | 69 | med |
| 75 | 0 | 0 | 17 | 1 | 141 | 55 | low |
| 183 | 11 | 5 | 13 | 7 | 12 | 39 | low |

# BREAKFAST CEREALS

| FOOD | SERVING SIZE | HOUSEHOLD MEASURE |
|------|------|------|
| Golden Grahams™, General Mills | 1 oz | ¾ cup |
| Grape-nuts™, Post | 8 oz | 1 cup |
| Grape-nuts™ Flakes, Post | 1.1 oz | ⅓ cup |
| Hi-Bran Weet-Bix®, regular | 1 oz | 1½ biscuits |
| Honey Smacks®, Kellogg's® | 1 oz | ¾ cup |
| Just Right®, Kellogg's® | 1½ oz | ¾ cup |
| Kashi® 7 Whole Grain Puffs | 0.7 oz | 1 cup |
| Life™, Quaker Oats | 1 oz | ¾ cup |
| Mini Wheats®, Blackcurrant, Kellogg's® | ¾ oz | 10 biscuits |
| Mini Wheats®, Wholewheat, Kellogg's® | ¾ oz | 13 biscuits |
| Muesli, gluten and wheat free with psyllium | 1½ oz | ½ cup |
| Muesli, mixed berry & apple | 1½ oz | ½ cup |
| Muesli, Morning Sun Apricot and Almond cereal | 1 oz | ⅓ cup |
| Muesli, Natural | 1 oz | ¼ cup |
| Muesli, Swiss Formula | 1 oz | ⅓ cup |
| Muesli, toasted, Purina | 1 oz | ⅓ cup |
| Muesli, yeast and wheat free | 1½ oz | ½ cup |
| Nutri-Grain®, Kellogg's® | ¾ oz | ½ cup |
| Oat bran, raw, unprocessed | 1 oz | ⅓ cup |
| Oats, rolled, raw | 1 oz | ⅓ cup |
| Oatmeal, multigrain, made with water | 1 oz | ⅓ cup |

© part of GI symbol program  ★ little or no carbs

| CALORIES | FAT (g) | SATURATED FAT (g) | CARBO-HYDRATE (g) | FIBER (g) | SODIUM (mg) | GI | LOW MED HIGH |
|---|---|---|---|---|---|---|---|
| 120 | 1 | 0 | 25 | 1 | 280 | 71 | high |
| 200 | 1 | 0 | 48 | 7 | 290 | 71 | high |
| 110 | 1 | 0 | 24 | 3 | 120 | 80 | high |
| 107 | 2 | 1 | 17 | 6 | 122 | 61 | med |
| 104 | 1 | 0 | 23 | 1 | 50 | 71 | high |
| 153 | 1 | 0 | 32 | 2 | 253 | 60 | med |
| 70 | 1 | 0 | 14 | 1 | 0 | 65 | med |
| 120 | 2 | 0 | 24 | 2 | 160 | 66 | med |
| 76 | 0 | 0 | 15 | 2 | 3 | 72 | high |
| 90 | 0 | 0 | 15 | 3 | 2 | 58 | med |
| 183 | 11 | 5 | 13 | 7 | 12 | 50 | low |
| 144 | 2 | 0 | 30 | 3 | 98 | 64 | med |
| 107 | 2 | 1 | 17 | 4 | 8 | 49 | low |
| 106 | 3 | 0 | 16 | 3 | 4 | 40 | low |
| 110 | 2 | 0 | 18 | 3 | 33 | 56 | med |
| 131 | 5 | 1 | 18 | 3 | 50 | 43 | low |
| 163 | 10 | 5 | 13 | 4 | 2 | 44 | low |
| 77 | 0 | 0 | 14 | 1 | 120 | 66 | med |
| 114 | 2 | 1 | 17 | 3 | 3 | 59 | med |
| 74 | 2 | 0 | 15 | 5 | 1 | 55 | low |
| 96 | 1 | 0 | 17 | 3 | 1 | 55 | low |

# BREAKFAST CEREALS

| FOOD | SERVING SIZE | HOUSEHOLD MEASURE |
|---|---|---|
| Oatmeal, instant, made with water | 6 oz | ¾ cup |
| Oatmeal, made from steel-cut oats with water | 6 oz | ¾ cup |
| Oatmeal, regular, made from oats with water | 6 oz | ¾ cup |
| President's Choice® Blue Menu™ Bran Flakes | 1 oz | ¾ cup |
| President's Choice® Blue Menu™ Fiber-First, multi-bran cereal | 1 oz | ½ cup |
| President's Choice® Blue Menu™ Granola Clusters, original, low-fat | 2 oz | ⅔ cup |
| President's Choice® Blue Menu™ Granola Clusters, Raisin Almond, low-fat | 2 oz | ⅔ cup |
| President's Choice® Blue Menu™ Multi-Grain Instant Oatmeal– Regular and Cinnamon & Spice | 1½ oz | 1 pouch |
| President's Choice® Blue Menu™ Omega-3 Granola Cereal | 2 oz | ⅔ cup |
| President's Choice® Blue Menu™ Soy Crunch Multi-Grain Cereal | 1.8 oz | ¾ cup |
| Soy Crunch Multi-Grain Cereal | 2 oz | ¾ cup |
| President's Choice® Blue Menu™ Steel-Cut Oats | 1¼ oz | ¼ cup |
| Puffed buckwheat | ¾ oz | ½ cup |
| Puffed Wheat, Quaker Oats | 1 oz | 1 cup |

@ part of GI symbol program   ★ little or no carbs

| CALORIES | FAT (g) | SATURATED FAT (g) | CARBO-HYDRATE (g) | FIBER (g) | SODIUM (mg) | GI | LOW MED HIGH |
|---|---|---|---|---|---|---|---|
| 101 | 3 | 0 | 18 | 3 | 0 | 82 | high |
| 101 | 3 | 0 | 18 | 3 | 0 | 52 | low |
| 101 | 3 | 0 | 18 | 3 | 0 | 58 | med |
| 110 | 1 | 0 | 24 | 5 | 190 | 65 | med |
| 110 | 1 | 0 | 23 | 13 | 270 | 55 | low |
| 220 | 3 | 1 | 40 | 4 | 55 | 63 | med |
| 220 | 3 | 1 | 40 | 3 | 50 | 70 | high |
| 170 | 3 | 1 | 26 | 6 | 160 | 55 | low |
| 230 | 6 | 1 | 37 | 5 | 65 | 43 | low |
| 230 | 3 | 1 | 40 | 4 | 130 | 47 | low |
| 230 | 3 | 1 | 36 | 4 | 130 | 47 | low |
| 150 | 2 | 0 | 29 | 4 | 0 | 51 | low |
| 67 | 1 | 0 | 15 | 1 | 0 | 65 | med |
| 102 | 1 | 0 | 21 | 3 | 1 | 67 | med |

# BREAKFAST CEREALS

| FOOD | SERVING SIZE | HOUSEHOLD MEASURE |
|------|------|------|
| Quick oats porridge | ¾ oz | ⅔ cup |
| Quick oats | 6 oz | 1 packet |
| Raisin Bran™, Kellogg's® | 1 oz | ½ cup |
| Red River Cereal, Maple Leaf Mills | 1 oz | ¼ cup |
| Rice Chex™, Nabisco | 1 oz | 1 cup |
| Rice Krispies™, Kellogg's® | 1.2 oz | 1¼ cups |
| Semolina, cooked | ¾ oz | ½ cup |
| Shredded Wheat™, Post | 1.6 oz | 2 biscuits |
| Special K™, Kellogg's® | 1.1 oz | 1 cup |
| Total™, General Mills | 1 oz | ¾ cup |
| Weetabix™ | 1 oz | 2 biscuits |

@ part of GI symbol program     ★ little or no carbs

| CALORIES | FAT (g) | SATURATED FAT (g) | CARBO-HYDRATE (g) | FIBER (g) | SODIUM (mg) | GI | LOW MED HIGH |
|---|---|---|---|---|---|---|---|
| 74 | 0 | 0 | 15 | 1 | 1 | 80 | high |
| 100 | 2 | 0 | 19 | 3 | 80 | 65 | med |
| 95 | 1 | 0 | 23 | 4 | 175 | 61 | med |
| 154 | 3 | 0 | 27 | 6 | 4 | 49 | low |
| 100 | 1 | 0 | 23 | 0 | 240 | 89 | high |
| 120 | 0 | 0 | 29 | 0 | 320 | 82 | high |
| 77 | 0 | 0 | 17 | 0 | 144 | 87 | high |
| 160 | 1 | 0 | 37 | 6 | 0 | 83 | high |
| 120 | 1 | 0 | 22 | 0 | 220 | 69 | med |
| 100 | 1 | 0 | 23 | 3 | 190 | 76 | high |
| 130 | 1 | 0 | 28 | 4 | 135 | 74 | high |

# CAKES & MUFFINS

| FOOD | SERVING SIZE | HOUSEHOLD MEASURE |
|------|------|------|
| 9 grain muffin | 1 oz | 2 muffins |
| Angel food cake | 1 oz | 1 small piece (⅛ of a 10-inch cake) |
| Apple berry crumble, commercially made | 3½ oz | 1 serving |
| Apple muffin, homemade | 1½ oz | ⅓ large |
| Apple, oat, raisin muffin | 1½ oz | 1 med. muffin |
| Apricot, coconut and honey muffin | 1½ oz | 1 med. muffin |
| Banana, oat and honey muffin | 1½ oz | 1 mufiin |
| Banana cake, homemade | 1½ oz | 1 thin slice (⅛ of a 10-inch cake) |
| Blueberry muffin | 1½ oz | 1 muffin |
| Blueberry muffin, commercially made | 1½ oz | ⅓ large |
| Bran muffin, commercially made | 1½ oz | ¾ average (2¾ inch diameter) |
| Carrot cake | 1 oz | 1 small piece |
| Carrot muffin, commercially made | 1½ oz | ⅓ large |
| Chocolate cake, made from packet mix with frosting, Betty Crocker® | 1 oz | 1 small piece (1/12 of a 6 x 2½ x 2½-inch cake) |
| Chocolate muffin | 1½ oz | ½ medium (2¾ inch diameter) |

@ part of GI symbol program  ★ little or no carbs

| CALORIES | FAT (g) | SATURATED FAT (g) | CARBO-HYDRATE (g) | FIBER (g) | SODIUM (mg) | GI | LOW MED HIGH |
|---|---|---|---|---|---|---|---|
| 79 | 2 | 0 | 11 | 2 | 86 | 43 | low |
| 77 | 1 | 0 | 15 | 0 | 137 | 67 | med |
| 300 | 15 | 6 | 40 | 2 | 3 | 41 | low |
| 129 | 6 | 1 | 17 | 0 | 150 | 46 | low |
| 277 | 6 | 2 | 36 | 2 | 290 | 54 | low |
| 248 | 11 | 3 | 34 | 1 | 280 | 60 | med |
| 114 | 5 | 2 | 17 | 2 | 197 | 65 | med |
| 138 | 7 | 2 | 17 | 1 | 210 | 51 | low |
| 167 | 8 | 2 | 22 | 1 | 134 | 59 | med |
| 127 | 6 | 1 | 17 | 0 | 150 | 59 | med |
| 120 | 5 | 2 | 16 | 2 | 207 | 60 | med |
| 103 | 6 | 2 | 12 | 1 | 158 | 36 | low |
| 127 | 6 | 1 | 17 | 0 | 150 | 62 | med |
| 110 | 6 | 3 | 14 | 0 | 91 | 38 | low |
| 150 | 7 | 1 | 18 | 1 | 93 | 53 | low |

# CAKES & MUFFINS

| FOOD | SERVING SIZE | HOUSEHOLD MEASURE |
|------|------|------|
| Chocolate butterscotch muffin | 1½ oz | 1 med. muffin |
| Croissant, plain | 1 oz | ½ average |
| Crumpet, white | 1½ oz | 1 round |
| Cupcake, strawberry-iced | 1 oz | ⅓ cupcake |
| Double chocolate muffin | 1½ oz | 1 muffin |
| Doughnut, cinnamon sugar | 1½ oz | 1 small |
| Doughnut, commercially made | 1½ oz | 1 doughnut |
| Egg custard | 4 oz | 1 small |
| Macaroons, coconut | 1 oz | 1 cookie |
| NutriSystem® Apple Strudel Scone | | 1 pastry |
| NutriSystem®, Blueberry Bran Muffin | 2 oz | 1 container |
| NutriSystem® Cranberry Orange Pastry | | 1 pastry |
| Oatmeal muffin, made from mix | 1½ oz | ⅓ large packet |
| Pancakes, buckwheat, gluten-free, packet mix | ¾ oz | 1 small |
| Pancakes, homemade | 3 oz | 2 pancakes |
| Pancakes, prepared from mix (6-inch diameter) | 2 oz | 1 medium |
| Pastry, puff | 1 oz | ⅛ sheet |
| Pound cake, Sara Lee® | 1 oz | 1 small slice |
| President's Choice® Blue Menu™ Apple Berry Crumble | 5¾ oz | 1 dessert |
| President's Choice® Blue Menu™ Apple Crisp | 4 oz | ⅛ dessert |

@ part of GI symbol program     ★ little or no carbs

| CALORIES | FAT (g) | SATURATED FAT (g) | CARBO-HYDRATE (g) | FIBER (g) | SODIUM (mg) | GI | LOW MED HIGH |
|---|---|---|---|---|---|---|---|
| 302 | 18 | 4 | 31 | 1 | 146 | 53 | low |
| 140 | 8 | 4 | 13 | 1 | 126 | 67 | med |
| 86 | 0 | 0 | 18 | 1 | 425 | 69 | med |
| 84 | 2 | 1 | 15 | 0 | 91 | 73 | high |
| 187 | 9 | 2 | 24 | 1 | 117 | 46 | low |
| 168 | 9 | 4 | 18 | 1 | 171 | 76 | high |
| 192 | 10 | 3 | 22 | 1 | 181 | 75 | high |
| 117 | 4 | 2 | 15 | 0 | 109 | 35 | low |
| 115 | 4 | 3 | 22 | 1 | 70 | 32 | low |
| 160 | 3 | 2 | 26 | 6 | 290 | 43 | low |
| 100 | 2 | 1 | 11 | 8 | 130 | 28 | low |
| 130 | 3 | 1 | 19 | 6 | 160 | 28 | low |
| 129 | 6 | 1 | 17 | 2 | 150 | 69 | med |
| 67 | 0 | 0 | 15 | 1 | 95 | 102 | high |
| 145 | 5 | 2 | 20 | 1 | 24 | 66 | med |
| 143 | 7 | 3 | 18 | 1 | 111 | 67 | med |
| 171 | 12 | 2 | 15 | 1 | 77 | 59 | med |
| 109 | 6 | 3 | 14 | 0 | 111 | 54 | low |
| 210 | 3 | 1 | 34 | 9 | 65 | 41 | low |
| 150 | 2 | 1 | 32 | 4 | 40 | 42 | low |

# CAKES & MUFFINS

| FOOD | SERVING SIZE | HOUSEHOLD MEASURE |
|------|------|------|
| President's Choice® Blue Menu™ Cranberry & Orange Soy Muffin | 2½ oz | 1 muffin |
| President's Choice® Blue Menu™ Doughnut, cake type | 1½ oz | 1 doughnut |
| President's Choice® Blue Menu™ Raisin Bran Flax Muffin | 2½ oz | 1 muffin |
| President's Choice® Blue Menu™ Raspberry & Pomegranate Whole Grain Muffin | 2½ oz | 1 muffin |
| President's Choice® Blue Menu™ Raspberry Coffee Cake | 1¾ oz | 1 thin slice (1/12 of a cake) |
| President's Choice® Blue Menu™ Whole Grain Banana & Prune Muffin | 2½ oz | 1 muffin |
| President's Choice® Blue Menu™ Whole Grain Carrots, Dates, Pineapples & Walnuts Muffin | 2½ oz | 1 muffin |
| President's Choice® Blue Menu™ Wild Blueberry 10-Grain Muffins | 2½ oz | 1 muffin |
| Sara Lee®, Apple and peach danish, light | 2 oz | 1 small slice |
| Sara Lee®, Apple blueberry muffin | 1½ oz | 1 med. muffin |
| Sara Lee®, Chocolate chip muffin | 1½ oz | 1 med. muffin |
| Sara Lee®, Chocolate honeycomb bavarian, light | 2 oz | 1 small piece |
| Scones, plain, made from packet mix | 1 oz | 1 small |

ⓖ part of GI symbol program  ★ little or no carbs

| CALORIES | FAT (g) | SATURATED FAT (g) | CARBO-HYDRATE (g) | FIBER (g) | SODIUM (mg) | GI | LOW MED HIGH |
|---|---|---|---|---|---|---|---|
| 180 | 2 | 1 | 29 | 3 | 260 | 48 | low |
| 181 | 10 | 3 | 23 | 1 | 171 | 76 | high |
| 200 | 3 | 1 | 33 | 5 | 210 | 51 | low |
| 190 | 2 | 1 | 33 | 5 | 280 | 58 | med |
| 160 | 6 | 1 | 22 | 2 | 160 | 50 | low |
| 190 | 2 | 1 | 39 | 3 | 190 | 39 | low |
| 180 | 3 | 1 | 34 | 4 | 210 | 53 | low |
| 220 | 3 | 1 | 39 | 3 | 190 | 57 | med |
| 174 | 8 | 5 | 20 | 2 | 60 | 50 | low |
| 248 | 16 | 2 | 33 | 2 | 245 | 49 | low |
| 284 | 16 | 2 | 30 | 2 | 150 | 52 | low |
| 202 | 14 | 8 | 16 | 1 | 149 | 31 | low |
| 110 | 3 | 1 | 17 | 1 | 182 | 92 | high |

# CAKES & MUFFINS

| FOOD | SERVING SIZE | HOUSEHOLD MEASURE |
|------|------|------|
| Sponge cake, plain, unfilled | 1 oz | 1 slice (3-inch diameter) |
| Vanilla cake, made from packet mix with vanilla frosting, Betty Crocker® | 1½ oz | 1 thin slice (¹⁄₂₄ of a 10-inch cake) |
| Waffle, plain | 1¼ oz | 1 square |
| Waffle, toasted | 1¼ oz | 1 square |

Ⓖ part of GI symbol program    ★ little or no carbs

| CALORIES | FAT (g) | SATURATED FAT (g) | CARBO-HYDRATE (g) | FIBER (g) | SODIUM (mg) | GI | LOW MED HIGH |
|---|---|---|---|---|---|---|---|
| 72 | 1 | 0 | 14 | 0 | 60 | 46 | low |
| 151 | 7 | 2 | 19 | 0 | 150 | 42 | low |
| 141 | 7 | 3 | 16 | 1 | 335 | 76 | high |
| 141 | 7 | 3 | 16 | 1 | 335 | 76 | high |

# CEREAL GRAINS

| FOOD | SERVING SIZE | HOUSEHOLD MEASURE |
|------|------|------|
| Barley, pearled, boiled | 2 oz | ⅓ cup |
| Buckwheat, boiled | 3 oz | ½ cup |
| Bulgur, cracked wheat | 3 oz | ⅓ cup |
| Millet, boiled | 2½ oz | ½ cup |
| Polenta (cornmeal), boiled | 6¾ oz | ¾ cup |
| Quinoa, boiled | 3½ oz | ½ cup |
| Rye, whole kernels | 1 oz | 2 tbsp |
| Semolina, cooked | 6 oz | ¾ cup |
| Whole-wheat kernels, boiled | 4 oz | ½ cup |

@ part of GI symbol program  ★ little or no carbs

| CALORIES | FAT (g) | SATURATED FAT (g) | CARBO-HYDRATE (g) | FIBER (g) | SODIUM (mg) | GI | LOW MED HIGH |
|---|---|---|---|---|---|---|---|
| 74 | 0 | 0 | 14 | 2 | 9 | 25 | low |
| 89 | 1 | 0 | 17 | 1 | 4 | 54 | low |
| 85 | 0 | 0 | 15 | 4 | 9 | 48 | low |
| 83 | 1 | 0 | 16 | 0 | 1 | 71 | high |
| 46 | 0 | 0 | 16 | 1 | 0 | 68 | med |
| 84 | 2 | 0 | 15 | 2 | 1 | 53 | low |
| 67 | 1 | 0 | 14 | 3 | 1 | 34 | low |
| 65 | 0 | 0 | 13 | 1 | 0 | 55 | low |
| 79 | 0 | 0 | 16 | 2 | 0 | 41 | low |

# COOKIES & CRACKERS

| FOOD | SERVING SIZE | HOUSEHOLD MEASURE |
|------|------|------|
| Apricot fruit cookies (97% fat free) | 1 oz | 1 cookie |
| Arrowroot, McCormicks's | ¾ oz | 4 cookies |
| Arrowroot plus, McCormicks's | ¾ oz | 4 cookies |
| Blueberry fruit cookies (97% fat free) | 1 oz | 1 cookie |
| Breton wheat crackers | 1 oz | 7 crackers |
| Chocolate chip cookies | 1 oz | 2 cookies |
| Corn Thins, puffed corn cakes, gluten-free | 1 oz | 4 slices |
| Digestives, plain | ¾ oz | 1½ cookies |
| Highland Oatcakes, Walker's | 1 oz | 2 oatcakes |
| Kavli Norwegian crispbread | ¾ oz | 4 crackers |
| Macaroons, coconut | 1 oz | 1 cookie |
| Milk Arrowroot | ¾ oz | 2 cookies |
| Oatmeal cookies | ¾ oz | 2 cookies |
| Premium Soda Crackers | 1 oz | 3 crackers |
| President's Choice® Blue Menu™ Ancient Grains Snack Crackers | ¾ oz | 10 crackers |
| President's Choice® Blue Menu™ Cranberry Orange Cookies | ¾ oz | 2 cookies |
| President's Choice® Blue Menu™ Crunchy Oat Cookies | ¾ oz | 2 cookies |
| President's Choice® Blue Menu™ Fat-free Fruit Bar, Apple | 1½ oz | 2 cookies |
| President's Choice® Blue Menu™ Fat-free Fruit Bar, Raspberry | 1½ oz | 2 cookies |

ⓖ part of GI symbol program ★ little or no carbs

| CALORIES | FAT (g) | SATURATED FAT (g) | CARBO- HYDRATE (g) | FIBER (g) | SODIUM (mg) | GI | LOW MED HIGH |
|---|---|---|---|---|---|---|---|
| 84 | 1 | 0 | 16 | 3 | 73 | 47 | low |
| 63 | 3 | 1 | 16 | 0 | 84 | 63 | med |
| 62 | 3 | 1 | 16 | 0 | 84 | 62 | med |
| 84 | 1 | 0 | 16 | 3 | 73 | 47 | low |
| 118 | 5 | 2 | 14 | 1 | 279 | 67 | med |
| 137 | 7 | 2 | 18 | 1 | 98 | 43 | low |
| 89 | 1 | 0 | 16 | 2 | 60 | 87 | high |
| 110 | 5 | 2 | 15 | 1 | 154 | 62 | med |
| 110 | 5 | 2 | 13 | 1 | 160 | 57 | med |
| 68 | 1 | 0 | 14 | 3 | 70 | 71 | high |
| 115 | 4 | 3 | 22 | 1 | 70 | 32 | low |
| 77 | 2 | 1 | 13 | 1 | 47 | 69 | med |
| 103 | 5 | 3 | 14 | 1 | 141 | 54 | low |
| 80 | 3 | 1 | 21 | 1 | 304 | 74 | high |
| 80 | 2 | 0 | 12 | 2 | 160 | 65 | med |
| 110 | 4 | 1 | 16 | 1 | 55 | 60 | med |
| 110 | 4 | 1 | 15 | 2 | 60 | 62 | med |
| 130 | 0 | 0 | 30 | 1 | 115 | 90 | high |
| 130 | 0 | 0 | 31 | 1 | 105 | 74 | high |

# COOKIES & CRACKERS

| FOOD | SERVING SIZE | HOUSEHOLD MEASURE |
|------|------|------|
| President's Choice® Blue Menu™ Fruit Bar, Fig | 1 ½ oz | 2 cookies |
| President's Choice® Blue Menu™ Fruit & Nut Whole Grain Soft Cookie | 1 ¼ oz | 1 cookie |
| President's Choice® Blue Menu™ Ginger and Lemon Cookies | ¾ oz | 2 cookies |
| President's Choice® Blue Menu™ Oatmeal Double Chocolate Soft Cookie | 1 ¼ oz | 1 cookie |
| President's Choice® Blue Menu™ Oatmeal Raisin Whole Grain Soft Cookie | 1 ¼ oz | 1 cookie |
| President's Choice® Blue Menu™ Wheat and Onion Snack Crackers | ¾ oz | 9 crackers |
| President's Choice® Blue Menu™ Wheat and Sesame Snack Crackers | ¾ oz | 9 crackers |
| President's Choice® Blue Menu™ Wheat Snack Crackers | ¾ oz | 9 crackers |
| President's Choice® Blue Menu™ Whole Wheat Fig Bar, 60% | 1 ½ oz | 2 cookies |
| Puffed crispbread | 1 oz | 3 crispbreads |
| Puffed Rice Cakes, white | ¾ oz | 2 rice cakes |
| Rice cracker, plain | ½ oz | 8 crackers |
| Rich tea biscuits | ¾ oz | 3 cookies |
| Rye crispbread | 1 oz | 3 crispbreads |
| Ryvita® Currant crispbread | ¾ oz | 1 ½ crispbreads |

| CALORIES | FAT (g) | SATURATED FAT (g) | CARBO-HYDRATE (g) | FIBER (g) | SODIUM (mg) | GI | LOW MED HIGH |
|---|---|---|---|---|---|---|---|
| 130 | 0 | 0 | 30 | 1 | 110 | 70 | high |
| 110 | 2 | 0 | 24 | 2 | 80 | 51 | low |
| 110 | 4 | 1 | 16 | 1 | 60 | 64 | med |
| 150 | 5 | 2 | 23 | 5 | 75 | 49 | low |
| 130 | 2 | 0 | 24 | 2 | 75 | 56 | med |
| 90 | 2 | 0 | 14 | 1 | 125 | 60 | med |
| 80 | 2 | 0 | 14 | 1 | 135 | 56 | med |
| 90 | 2 | 0 | 14 | 1 | 135 | 65 | med |
| 130 | 0 | 0 | 29 | 2 | 110 | 72 | high |
| 95 | 1 | 0 | 18 | 1 | 137 | 81 | high |
| 75 | 1 | 0 | 15 | 1 | 1 | 82 | high |
| 60 | 1 | 0 | 11 | 0 | 78 | 91 | high |
| 111 | 4 | 2 | 18 | 1 | 116 | 55 | low |
| 70 | 0 | 0 | 28 | 5 | 75 | 63 | med |
| 82 | 1 | 0 | 16 | 3 | 5 | 66 | med |

# COOKIES & CRACKERS

| FOOD | SERVING SIZE | HOUSEHOLD MEASURE |
|------|--------------|-------------------|
| Ryvita® Original Rye crispbread | ¾ oz | 2 crispbreads |
| ⓖ Ryvita® Pumpkin Seeds and Oats crispbread | 1 oz | 2 crispbreads |
| Ryvita® Sesame Rye crispbread | ¾ oz | 2 crispbreads |
| ⓖ Ryvita® Sunflower Seeds and Oats crispbread | 1 oz | 2 crispbreads |
| Shortbread biscuits, plain | 1 oz | 2 cookies |
| Shredded Wheat cookies | ¾ oz | 2 cookies |
| Snack Right® Fruit Roll, Spicy Apple and Raisin | ¾ oz | 1 cookie |
| Snack Right® Fruit Slice, Apricot | ¾ oz | 2 slices |
| Snack Right® Fruit Slice, Mango and Passionfruit | ¾ oz | 2 slices |
| Snack Right® Fruit Slice, Mixed Berry | ¾ oz | 2 slices |
| Snack Right® Fruit Slice, Raisin | 1 oz | 2 slices |
| Snack Right® Fruit Slice, Raisin and Chocolate | 1 oz | 2 slices |
| Spicy Apple fruit cookies (97% fat free) | 1 oz | 1 cookie |
| Sticky Date fruit cookies (97% fat free) | 1 oz | 1 cookie |
| Stoned Wheat Thins | 1 oz | 10 crackers |
| Vanilla wafer cookies, plain | 1 oz | 2 cookies |
| Water cracker | 1 oz | 7 crackers |
| Wheat cracker, plain | 1 oz | 3 crackers |
| Zesty Ginger fruit cookies (97% fat free) | 1 oz | 1 cookie |

ⓖ part of GI symbol program  ★ little or no carbs

| CALORIES | FAT (g) | SATURATED FAT (g) | CARBO-HYDRATE (g) | FIBER (g) | SODIUM (mg) | GI | LOW MED HIGH |
|---|---|---|---|---|---|---|---|
| 70 | 0 | 0 | 13 | 3 | 68 | 69 | med |
| 98 | 3 | 1 | 14 | 4 | 100 | 48 | low |
| 74 | 1 | 0 | 12 | 3 | 84 | 64 | med |
| 92 | 2 | 0 | 14 | 4 | 96 | 48 | low |
| 119 | 6 | 3 | 15 | 1 | 110 | 64 | med |
| 102 | 4 | 2 | 15 | 1 | 94 | 62 | med |
| 66 | 1 | 0 | 12 | 1 | 40 | 45 | low |
| 72 | 1 | 0 | 15 | 1 | 32 | 52 | low |
| 75 | 1 | 0 | 16 | 1 | 30 | 49 | low |
| 74 | 1 | 0 | 16 | 1 | 31 | 50 | low |
| 82 | 1 | 0 | 17 | 1 | 35 | 48 | low |
| 100 | 2 | 1 | 18 | 1 | 33 | 45 | low |
| 84 | 1 | 0 | 16 | 3 | 73 | 47 | low |
| 84 | 1 | 0 | 16 | 3 | 73 | 47 | low |
| 130 | 6 | 2 | 19 | 1 | 226 | 67 | med |
| 132 | 1 | 1 | 16 | 0 | 17 | 77 | high |
| 94 | 2 | 1 | 15 | 1 | 125 | 63 | med |
| 124 | 4 | 2 | 18 | 1 | 181 | 70 | high |
| 84 | 1 | 0 | 16 | 3 | 73 | 47 | low |

# DAIRY PRODUCTS: CHEESES

| FOOD | SERVING SIZE | HOUSEHOLD MEASURE |
|---|---|---|
| Brie | 1 oz | 2 tbsp |
| Camembert | 1 oz | 2 tbsp |
| Cheddar | 1 oz | 1½ slices |
| Cheddar, 25% reduced fat | 1 oz | 1½ slices |
| Cheddar, 50% reduced fat | 1 oz | 1½ slices |
| Cheddar, low fat | 1 oz | 1½ slices |
| Cheddar, reduced salt | 1 oz | 1½ slices |
| Cheese spread, cheddar | 1 oz | 1½ tbsp |
| Cheese spread, cheddar, reduced fat | 1 oz | 1½ tbsp |
| Cottage cheese | 1 oz | 2 tbsp |
| Cottage cheese, low fat | 1 oz | 2 tbsp |
| Cream cheese | 1 oz | 1½ tbsp |
| Cream cheese dip | 1 oz | 1½ tbsp |
| Cream cheese, reduced fat | 1 oz | 1½ tbsp |
| Feta | 1 oz | 2 tbsp |
| Feta, low salt | 1 oz | 2 tbsp |
| Feta, reduced fat | 1 oz | 2 tbsp |
| Mozzarella | 1 oz | 1½ slices |
| Mozzarella, reduced fat | 1 oz | 1½ slices |
| Parmesan | 1 oz | ⅓ cup |
| Ricotta | 1 oz | 2 tbsp |
| Ricotta, reduced fat | 1 oz | 2 tbsp |
| Soy cheese | 1 oz | 1½ slices |

@ part of GI symbol program   ★ little or no carbs

| CALORIES | FAT (g) | SATURATED FAT (g) | CARBO-HYDRATE (g) | FIBER (g) | SODIUM (mg) | GI | LOW MED HIGH |
|---|---|---|---|---|---|---|---|
| 102 | 9 | 6 | 0 | 0 | 182 | ★ | |
| 93 | 8 | 5 | 0 | 0 | 195 | ★ | |
| 122 | 10 | 7 | 0 | 0 | 197 | ★ | |
| 99 | 7 | 5 | 0 | 0 | 216 | ★ | |
| 80 | 5 | 3 | 0 | 0 | 207 | ★ | |
| 61 | 2 | 1 | 0 | 0 | 198 | ★ | |
| 123 | 11 | 7 | 0 | 0 | 111 | ★ | |
| 87 | 7 | 5 | 1 | 0 | 435 | ★ | |
| 72 | 5 | 3 | 2 | 0 | 480 | ★ | |
| 37 | 2 | 1 | 1 | 0 | 95 | ★ | |
| 27 | 0 | 0 | 1 | 0 | 39 | ★ | |
| 102 | 10 | 6 | 1 | 0 | 126 | ★ | |
| 76 | 7 | 4 | 3 | 0 | 204 | ★ | |
| 58 | 5 | 3 | 1 | 0 | 102 | ★ | |
| 84 | 7 | 5 | 0 | 0 | 321 | ★ | |
| 113 | 10 | 7 | 0 | 0 | 66 | ★ | |
| 70 | 4 | 3 | 0 | 0 | 330 | ★ | |
| 91 | 7 | 4 | 0 | 0 | 113 | ★ | |
| 86 | 5 | 4 | 0 | 0 | 174 | ★ | |
| 133 | 10 | 6 | 0 | 0 | 432 | ★ | |
| 44 | 3 | 2 | 0 | 0 | 59 | ★ | |
| 38 | 3 | 2 | 0 | 0 | 56 | ★ | |
| 95 | 8 | 1 | 0 | 0 | 180 | ★ | |

# DAIRY PRODUCTS: ICE CREAM, CUSTARDS, PUDDINGS & DESSERTS

| FOOD | SERVING SIZE | HOUSEHOLD MEASURE |
|------|------|------|
| Chocolate Mousse, Nestlé® | 3 oz | 1½ containers |
| Chocolate Mousse, Diet, Nestlé® | 2¾ oz | ⅓ cup |
| Chocolate pudding, instant, made from packet with full fat milk | 4½ oz | ⅙ packet |
| Chocolate shake, low fat chocolate soft serve with skim milk and malted milk powder | 10 fl oz | 1 large cup |
| Crème Caramel, Diet, Nestlé® | 4 oz | 1 tub |
| Custard, homemade from milk, wheat starch and sugar | 2 oz | ¼ cup |
| Custard, low fat | 4 fl oz | ½ cup |
| Frutia, low fat frozen fruit dessert, Mango, Weis | 2 fl oz | ⅒ tub |
| Gelato, sucrose-free, chocolate | 2 oz | 1 scoop |
| Gelato, sucrose-free, vanilla | 2 oz | 1 scoop |
| Icecream, light creamy low fat, chocolate | 2½ fl oz | 1½ scoops |
| Icecream, light creamy low fat, English toffee | 2½ fl oz | 1½ scoops |
| Icecream, light creamy low fat, mango | 2½ fl oz | 1½ scoops |
| Icecream, light creamy low fat, vanilla | 2½ fl oz | 1½ scoops |
| Icecream, low carbohydrate, chocolate | 3½ fl oz | 2 scoops |

@ part of GI symbol program   ★ little or no carbs

| CALORIES | FAT (g) | SATURATED FAT (g) | CARBO-HYDRATE (g) | FIBER (g) | SODIUM (mg) | GI | LOW MED HIGH |
|---|---|---|---|---|---|---|---|
| 98 | 2 | 2 | 15 | 0 | 45 | 37 | low |
| 100 | 5 | 2 | 13 | 0 | 113 | 31 | low |
| 133 | 4 | 3 | 20 | 0 | 240 | 47 | low |
| 242 | 4 | 2 | 38 | 0 | 160 | 21 | low |
| 76 | 1 | 1 | 23 | 0 | 85 | 33 | low |
| 83 | 2 | 1 | 14 | 0 | 29 | 43 | low |
| 102 | 1 | 1 | 18 | 0 | 59 | 38 | low |
| 73 | 0 | 0 | 17 | 0 | 3 | 42 | low |
| 84 | 3 | 2 | 14 | 0 | 34 | 37 | low |
| 76 | 2 | 1 | 14 | 0 | 34 | 39 | low |
| 104 | 1 | 1 | 16 | 0 | 35 | 27 | low |
| 74 | 1 | 1 | 14 | 1 | 30 | 27 | low |
| 72 | 1 | 1 | 13 | 1 | 25 | 30 | low |
| 93 | 1 | 1 | 17 | 1 | 38 | 36 | low |
| 61 | 2 | 1 | 5 | 5 | 44 | 32 | low |

# DAIRY PRODUCTS: ICE CREAM, CUSTARDS, PUDDINGS & DESSERTS

| FOOD | SERVING SIZE | HOUSEHOLD MEASURE |
|------|------|------|
| Icecream, regular, full fat, average of several types | 2½ fl oz | 1½ scoops |
| Icecream, Sara Lee®, full fat, French Vanilla | 1¾ fl oz | 1 scoop |
| Icecream, Sara Lee®, full fat, Ultra Chocolate | 1¾ fl oz | 1 scoop |
| Low fat chocolate soft serve ice cream | 2 oz | 1 scoop |
| Low fat chocolate soft serve eaten with a plain cone | 4 oz | 1 cone |
| Low fat chocolate soft serve eaten with a waffle cone | 4 oz | 1 cone |
| Nestlé® Citrus Flavor Mousse dessert mix | 1 oz | 2 scoops |
| President's Choice® Blue Menu™ Frozen yogurt, Mochaccino | 4 fl oz | ½ cup |
| President's Choice® Blue Menu™ Frozen yogurt, Strawberry Banana | 4 fl oz | ½ cup |
| President's Choice® Blue Menu™ Frozen yogurt, Vanilla | 4 fl oz | ½ cup |
| Tapioca pudding, boiled, with milk | 4 oz | ½ cup |
| Vanilla frozen yogurt | 2½ oz | ½ cup |
| Vanilla pudding, instant, made from packet mix with full fat milk | 3 oz | ⅛ packet prepared |

Ⓖ part of GI symbol program   ★ little or no carbs

| CALORIES | FAT (g) | SATURATED FAT (g) | CARBO-HYDRATE (g) | FIBER (g) | SODIUM (mg) | GI | LOW MED HIGH |
|---|---|---|---|---|---|---|---|
| 138 | 8 | 5 | 15 | 0 | 44 | 47 | low |
| 202 | 13 | 9 | 18 | 0 | 41 | 38 | low |
| 196 | 12 | 8 | 19 | 0 | 53 | 37 | low |
| 51 | 0.4 | 0.3 | 9 | 0 | 28 | 24 | low |
| 100 | 1.7 | 1.3 | 20 | 1 | 53 | 44 | low |
| 158 | 1.7 | 1.3 | 28 | 1 | 53 | 55 | low |
| 110 | 5 | 3 | 14 | 0 | 84 | 47 | low |
| 120 | 2 | 1 | 21 | 0 | 65 | 51 | low |
| 110 | 2 | 1 | 20 | 0 | 60 | 55 | low |
| 110 | 2 | 1 | 21 | 0 | 65 | 46 | low |
| 125 | 4 | 2 | 18 | 0 | 57 | 81 | high |
| 114 | 4 | 2 | 17 | 0 | 63 | 46 | low |
| 103 | 3 | 2 | 15 | 0 | 190 | 40 | low |

# DAIRY PRODUCTS: ICE CREAM, CUSTARDS, PUDDINGS & DESSERTS

| FOOD | SERVING SIZE | HOUSEHOLD MEASURE |
|------|------|------|
| Vanilla pudding, Sustagen®, powdered mix | 1 oz | ½ scoop |
| Wild Berry, non-dairy, frozen fruit dessert | 1¾ fl oz | 1 scoop |
| Yoplait Le Rice, dairy rice desserts, Apple Cinnamon | 3 oz | ½ container |
| Yoplait Le Rice, dairy rice desserts, Apricot and Almond Muesli | 3 oz | ½ container |
| Yoplait Le Rice, dairy rice desserts, Caramel | 3 oz | ½ container |
| Yoplait Le Rice, dairy rice desserts, Classic Vanilla | 3 oz | ½ container |
| Yoplait Le Rice, dairy rice desserts, Forest Berries | 3 oz | ½ container |
| Yoplait Le Rice, dairy rice desserts, Raspberry and Apple | 3 oz | ½ container |
| Yoplait Le Rice, dairy rice desserts, Strawberry | 3 oz | ½ container |
| Yoplait Le Rice, dairy rice desserts, Tropical Mango | 3 oz | ½ container |

@ part of GI symbol program     ★ little or no carbs

| CALORIES | FAT (g) | SATURATED FAT (g) | CARBO-HYDRATE (g) | FIBER (g) | SODIUM (mg) | GI | LOW MED HIGH |
|---|---|---|---|---|---|---|---|
| 139 | 6 | 1 | 18 | 0 | 288 | 27 | low |
| 48 | 0 | 0 | 12 | 0 | 10 | 59 | med |
| 104 | 2 | 1 | 19 | 0 | 52 | 52 | low |
| 105 | 2 | 1 | 19 | 0 | 64 | 45 | low |
| 105 | 2 | 1 | 19 | 0 | 53 | 41 | low |
| 105 | 2 | 1 | 19 | 0 | 59 | 36 | low |
| 99 | 2 | 1 | 17 | 0 | 64 | 45 | low |
| 104 | 2 | 1 | 19 | 0 | 55 | 52 | low |
| 104 | 2 | 1 | 18 | 0 | 53 | 54 | low |
| 103 | 2 | 1 | 19 | 0 | 51 | 54 | low |

# DAIRY PRODUCTS: MILK & ALTERNATIVES

| FOOD | SERVING SIZE | HOUSEHOLD MEASURE |
|---|---|---|
| Blue Diamond Refrigerated Unsweetened Vanilla Breeze (almond beverage) | 8 fl oz | 1 cup |
| Blue Diamond Unsweetened Chocolate Breeze (almond beverage) | 8 fl oz | 1 cup |
| Blue Diamond Unsweetened Original Breeze (almond beverage) | 8 fl oz | 1 cup |
| Blue Diamond Unsweetened Vanilla Breeze (almond beverage) | 8 fl oz | 1 cup |
| Chocolate-flavored, low fat milk | 8½ fl oz | 1 cup |
| Chocolate-flavored milk | 5¼ fl oz | ½ small carton |
| Condensed milk, sweetened, full fat | 1 oz | 1 tbsp |
| Lite White, reduced fat (1.4%) milk | 8 fl oz | 1 cup |
| Milk (3.6% fat) | 8 fl oz | 1 cup |
| Milk, calcium-enriched, low fat (0.1%) | 8 fl oz | 1 cup |
| Milk, reduced fat | 8 fl oz | 1 cup |
| Milk with omega-3 | 8½ fl oz | 1 cup |
| Mocha-flavored, low fat milk | 8½ fl oz | 1 cup |
| Mocha-flavored milk | 8½ fl oz | 1 cup |
| Probiotic fermented milk drink with *Lactobacillus casei* | 2¼ fl oz | 1 std serve |
| Skim, low fat (0.1%) milk | 8 fl oz | 1 cup |

★ little or no carbs  ■ high in saturated fat

| CALORIES | FAT (g) | SATURATED FAT (g) | CARBO-HYDRATE (g) | FIBER (g) | SODIUM (mg) | GI | LOW MED HIGH |
|---|---|---|---|---|---|---|---|
| 40 | 3 | 0 | 2 | 1 | 180 | 23 | low |
| 45 | 3.5 | 0 | 3 | 1 | 180 | 23 | low |
| 40 | 3 | 0 | 2 | 1 | 180 | 23 | low |
| 40 | 3 | 0 | 2 | 1 | 180 | 23 | low |
| 158 | 3 | 2 | 25 | 0 | 152 | 27 | low |
| 120 | 4 | 3 | 15 | 0 | 69 | 37 | low |
| 82 | 2 | 2 | 14 | 0 | 27 | 61 | med |
| 127 | 4 | 2 | 14 | 0 | 128 | 30 | low |
| 168 | 10 | 7 | 12 | 0 | 106 | 27 | low |
| 121 | 0 | 0 | 17 | 0 | 173 | 34 | low |
| 122 | 5 | 3 | 11 | 0 | 100 | 30 | low |
| 134 | 3 | 0 | 16 | 0 | 174 | 27 | low |
| 133 | 1 | 0 | 17 | 0 | 143 | 27 | low |
| 206 | 9 | 6 | 24 | 0 | 98 | 32 | low |
| 52 | 0 | 0 | 12 | 0 | 10 | 46 | low |
| 89 | 0 | 0 | 12 | 0 | 128 | 32 | low |

# DAIRY PRODUCTS: MILK & ALTERNATIVES

| FOOD | SERVING SIZE | HOUSEHOLD MEASURE |
|------|------|------|
| @ So Natural Calciforte, soy milk, calcium-enriched, full fat | 8 fl oz | 1 cup |
| So Natural Light, soy milk, reduced fat, calcium-fortified | 8 fl oz | 1 cup |
| So Natural Original, soy milk, full fat (3%) | 8 fl oz | 1 cup |
| Strawberry-flavored milk | 5¼ fl oz | ½ small carton |
| Vitasoy® Light Original, soy milk | 8 fl oz | 1 cup |
| Vitasoy® Lush, chocolate, reduced fat soy milk | 8 fl oz | 1 cup |
| Vitasoy® Lush, vanilla, reduced fat soy milk | 8 fl oz | 1 cup |
| Vitasoy® Organic soy milk | 8 fl oz | 1 cup |
| Vitasoy® Premium Calci Plus® High Fiber, soy milk, 98.5% fat free | 8 fl oz | 1 cup |
| Vitasoy® Soy Milky, regular, soy milk | 8 fl oz | 1 cup |
| Vitasoy® Soy Milky, lite, soy milk | 8 fl oz | 1 cup |
| Vitasoy® Premium Calci Plus®, soy milk | 8 fl oz | 1 cup |
| Vitasoy®, rice milk, calcium-enriched | 8 fl oz | 1 cup |
| Yakult®, fermented milk drink with *Lactobacillus casei* | 2.2 fl oz | 1 bottle |
| Yakult® Light, fermented milk drink with *Lactobacillus casei* | 2.2 fl oz | 1 bottle |

@ part of GI symbol program     ★ little or no carbs

| CALORIES | FAT (g) | SATURATED FAT (g) | CARBO-HYDRATE (g) | FIBER (g) | SODIUM (mg) | GI | LOW MED HIGH |
|---|---|---|---|---|---|---|---|
| 171 | 7 | 1 | 19 | 1 | 233 | 40 | low |
| 105 | 1 | 0 | 14 | 1 | 98 | 44 | low |
| 150 | 7 | 1 | 19 | 1 | 225 | 44 | low |
| 116 | 4 | 3 | 15 | 0 | 65 | 37 | low |
| 53 | 2 | 0 | 8 | 0 | 80 | 45 | low |
| 139 | 4 | 1 | 19 | 1 | 218 | 31 | low |
| 128 | 4 | 1 | 16 | 1 | 165 | 31 | low |
| 120 | 4 | 1 | 16 | 3 | 30 | 43 | low |
| 121 | 4 | 1 | 14 | 4 | 110 | 16 | low |
| 132 | 8 | 1 | 8 | 1 | 225 | 21 | low |
| 95 | 4 | 1 | 7 | 1 | 225 | 17 | low |
| 160 | 8 | 2 | 15 | 1 | 120 | 24 | low |
| 123 | 3 | 0 | 24 | 2 | 157 | 79 | high |
| 52 | 0 | 0 | 12 | 0 | 10 | 46 | low |
| 35 | 0 | 0 | 9 | 2 | 10 | 36 | low |

# DAIRY PRODUCTS: YOGURT

| FOOD | SERVING SIZE | HOUSEHOLD MEASURE |
|------|------|------|
| ⓖ Nestlé® All Natural 99% Fat Free Plain Natural | 7 oz | I container |
| ⓖ Nestlé® All Natural Apple & Cinnamon | 7 oz | I container |
| ⓖ Nestlé® All Natural Black Cherry | 7 oz | I container |
| ⓖ Nestlé® All Natural Light Apricot | 7 oz | I container |
| ⓖ Nestlé® All Natural Light Tropical Fruit Salad | 7 oz | I container |
| ⓖ Nestlé® All Natural Light Vanilla | 7 oz | I container |
| ⓖ Nestlé® All Natural Passionfruit | 7 oz | I container |
| ⓖ Nestlé® All Natural Peaches & Cream | 7 oz | I container |
| ⓖ Nestlé® All Natural Peach Mango | 7 oz | I container |
| ⓖ Nestlé® diet, low fat, all flavors | 7 oz | I container |
| Yogurt, low fat, natural | 7 oz | I container |
| Yogurt, low fat, no added sugar, vanilla or fruit | 7 oz | I container |
| Yoplait Lite Apricot yogurt | 3½ oz | ½ container |
| Yoplait Lite Berry Bliss yogurt | 3½ oz | ½ container |
| Yoplait Lite Blueberry Crème yogurt | 3½ oz | ½ container |
| Yoplait Lite Blueberry yogurt | 3½ oz | ½ container |
| Yoplait Lite Creamy Vanilla yogurt | 3½ oz | ½ container |

ⓖ part of GI symbol program   ★ little or no carbs

| CALORIES | FAT (g) | SATURATED FAT (g) | CARBO-HYDRATE (g) | FIBER (g) | SODIUM (mg) | GI | LOW MED HIGH |
|---|---|---|---|---|---|---|---|
| 136 | 2 | 2 | 17 | 0 | 134 | 14 | low |
| 83 | 0 | 0 | 11 | 0 | 90 | 30 | low |
| 83 | 0 | 0 | 11 | 0 | 87 | 55 | low |
| 83 | 0 | 0 | 11 | 0 | 87 | 49 | low |
| 84 | 0 | 0 | 11 | 0 | 87 | 38 | low |
| 80 | 0 | 0 | 11 | 0 | 88 | 37 | low |
| 82 | 0 | 0 | 11 | 0 | 90 | 47 | low |
| 82 | 0 | 0 | 11 | 0 | 90 | 28 | low |
| 85 | 0 | 0 | 12 | 0 | 88 | 33 | low |
| 82 | 0 | 0 | 11 | 0 | 88 | 19–21 | low |
| 111 | 0 | 0 | 15 | 0 | 153 | 35 | low |
| 156 | 1 | 0 | 17 | 0 | 230 | 20 | low |
| 89 | 1 | 1 | 16 | 0 | 72 | 27 | low |
| 90 | 1 | 1 | 16 | 0 | 77 | 25 | low |
| 95 | 1 | 1 | 17 | 0 | 78 | 25 | low |
| 94 | 1 | 1 | 17 | 0 | 75 | 25 | low |
| 94 | 1 | 1 | 17 | 0 | 76 | 27 | low |

# DAIRY PRODUCTS: YOGURT

| FOOD | SERVING SIZE | HOUSEHOLD MEASURE |
|---|---|---|
| Yoplait Lite Field Strawberries yogurt | 3½ oz | ½ container |
| Yoplait Lite French Cheesecake yogurt | 3½ oz | ½ container |
| Yoplait Lite Fruit Salad yogurt | 3½ oz | ½ container |
| Yoplait Lite Lemon Meringue yogurt | 3½ oz | ½ container |
| Yoplait Lite Mango Passion yogurt | 3½ oz | ½ container |
| Yoplait Lite Mango yogurt | 3½ oz | ½ container |
| Yoplait Lite Passionfruit yogurt | 3½ oz | ½ container |
| Yoplait Lite Peach Mango yogurt | 3½ oz | ½ container |
| Yoplait Lite Rhubarb Custard yogurt | 3½ oz | ½ container |
| Yoplait Lite Strawberry yogurt | 3½ oz | ½ container |
| Yoplait Lite Tropical Mango yogurt | 3½ oz | ½ container |
| Yoplait Lite Tropical yogurt | 3½ oz | ½ container |
| Yoplait Lite Vanilla Strawberry yogurt | 3½ oz | ½ container |
| Yoplait No Fat Apple Pie yogurt | 7 oz | 1 container |
| Yoplait No Fat Apricot yogurt | 7 oz | 1 container |
| Yoplait No Fat Banana Creamy Honey yogurt | 7 oz | 1 container |
| Yoplait No Fat Berry Brulée yogurt | 7 oz | 1 container |
| Yoplait No Fat Berry Crëme yogurt | 7 oz | 1 container |

ⓖ part of GI symbol program   ★ little or no carbs

| CALORIES | FAT (g) | SATURATED FAT (g) | CARBO-HYDRATE (g) | FIBER (g) | SODIUM (mg) | GI | LOW MED HIGH |
|---|---|---|---|---|---|---|---|
| 94 | 1 | 1 | 17 | 0 | 85 | 25 | low |
| 100 | 1 | 1 | 18 | 0 | 76 | 27 | low |
| 92 | 1 | 1 | 17 | 0 | 78 | 32 | low |
| 90 | 1 | 1 | 16 | 0 | 101 | 27 | low |
| 93 | 1 | 1 | 17 | 0 | 77 | 37 | low |
| 94 | 1 | 1 | 17 | 0 | 76 | 37 | low |
| 89 | 1 | 1 | 15 | 0 | 76 | 37 | low |
| 92 | 1 | 1 | 17 | 0 | 78 | 37 | low |
| 95 | 1 | 1 | 17 | 0 | 87 | 27 | low |
| 90 | 1 | 1 | 16 | 0 | 81 | 25 | low |
| 94 | 1 | 1 | 17 | 0 | 76 | 32 | low |
| 90 | 1 | 1 | 16 | 0 | 82 | 37 | low |
| 93 | 1 | 1 | 17 | 0 | 79 | 25 | low |
| 99 | 0 | 0 | 14 | 0 | 154 | 18 | low |
| 100 | 0 | 0 | 14 | 0 | 162 | 20 | low |
| 102 | 0 | 0 | 15 | 0 | 148 | 18 | low |
| 100 | 0 | 0 | 14 | 0 | 160 | 18 | low |
| 98 | 0 | 0 | 14 | 0 | 158 | 16 | low |

# DAIRY PRODUCTS: YOGURT

| FOOD | SERVING SIZE | HOUSEHOLD MEASURE |
|------|------|------|
| Yoplait No Fat Black Cherry yogurt | 7 oz | I container |
| Yoplait No Fat Boysenberry yogurt | 7 oz | I container |
| Yoplait No Fat French Cheesecake yogurt | 11 oz | 1½ containers |
| Yoplait No Fat French Vanilla yogurt | 7 oz | I container |
| Yoplait No Fat Mango yogurt | 7 oz | I container |
| Yoplait No Fat Passionfruit Crëme yogurt | 7 oz | I container |
| Yoplait No Fat Passionfruit yogurt | 7 oz | I container |
| Yoplait No Fat Peach Crëme yogurt | 7 oz | I container |
| Yoplait No Fat Peach Mango yogurt | 7 oz | I container |
| Yoplait No Fat Raspberry yogurt | 7 oz | I container |
| Yoplait No Fat Strawberry yogurt | 7 oz | I container |
| Yoplait No Fat Tropical yogurt | 7 oz | I container |

@ part of GI symbol program    ★ little or no carbs

| CALORIES | FAT (g) | SATURATED FAT (g) | CARBO-HYDRATE (g) | FIBER (g) | SODIUM (mg) | GI | LOW MED HIGH |
|---|---|---|---|---|---|---|---|
| 97 | 0 | 0 | 14 | 0 | 150 | 16 | low |
| 96 | 0 | 0 | 13 | 0 | 168 | 16 | low |
| 153 | 0 | 0 | 14 | 0 | 225 | 18 | low |
| 92 | 0 | 0 | 14 | 0 | 150 | 20 | low |
| 85 | 0 | 0 | 14 | 0 | 160 | 20 | low |
| 99 | 0 | 0 | 14 | 0 | 192 | 18 | low |
| 99 | 0 | 0 | 14 | 0 | 192 | 20 | low |
| 98 | 0 | 0 | 14 | 0 | 154 | 18 | low |
| 96 | 0 | 0 | 13 | 0 | 152 | 20 | low |
| 96 | 0 | 0 | 14 | 0 | 158 | 16 | low |
| 93 | 0 | 0 | 13 | 0 | 152 | 16 | low |
| 97 | 0 | 0 | 14 | 0 | 178 | 20 | low |

# FRUIT

| FOOD | SERVING SIZE | HOUSEHOLD MEASURE |
|------|------|------|
| Apple | 4 oz | 1 small |
| Apple, canned, solid pack without juice | 4½ oz | ½ cup |
| Apple, dried | 1 oz | 4 rings |
| Apricots | 6 oz | 2 large |
| Apricots, canned, in light syrup | 4½ oz | ½ cup |
| Apricots, dried | 1 oz | 10 pieces |
| Apricot halves, canned in fruit juice | 4½ oz | ½ cup |
| Avocado | 2¾ oz | ⅓ average |
| Banana | 3 oz | 1 small |
| Breadfruit | 2 oz | ¼ cup |
| Blueberries, wild | 3½ oz | ½ cup |
| Cantaloupe | 12 oz | 2 cups |
| Cherries, dark | 4½ oz | 1 cup |
| Cherries, dried, tart | 1 ½ oz | ¼ cup |
| Cherries, frozen, tart | 3 ½ oz | ⅔ cup |
| Cherries, raw, sour | 5 oz | 1 cup |
| Cherries, sour, pitted, canned | 4 oz | ½ cup |
| Cranberries, dried, sweetened | ¾ oz | 3 tbsp |
| Custard apple | 3 oz | ¼ large custard apple |
| Dates, Arabic, vacuum-packed | 2 oz | 3 medium |
| Dates, pitted | 1 oz | 5 average |
| Figs | 2 oz | 1 medium fig |

@ part of GI symbol program   ★ little or no carbs

| CALORIES | FAT (g) | SATURATED FAT (g) | CARBO- HYDRATE (g) | FIBER (g) | SODIUM (mg) | GI | LOW MED HIGH |
|---|---|---|---|---|---|---|---|
| 58 | 0 | 0 | 13 | 2 | 1 | 38 | low |
| 50 | 0 | 0 | 10 | 2 | 6 | 42 | low |
| 69 | 0 | 0 | 16 | 2 | 1 | 29 | low |
| 70 | 0 | 0 | 13 | 4 | 3 | 57 | med |
| 72 | 0 | 0 | 16 | 2 | 3 | 64 | med |
| 75 | 0 | 0 | 16 | 3 | 13 | 30 | low |
| 58 | 0 | 0 | 12 | 1 | 7 | 51 | low |
| 171 | 18 | 4 | 0 | 1 | 2 | ★ | |
| 73 | 0 | 0 | 16 | 2 | 1 | 52 | low |
| 57 | 0 | 0 | 26 | 3 | 1 | 62 | med |
| 45 | 0 | 0 | 9 | 4 | 0 | 53 | low |
| 80 | 0 | 0 | 16 | 3 | 34 | 65 | med |
| 73 | 0 | 0 | 15 | 2 | 1 | 63 | med |
| 153 | 0 | 0 | 30 | 3 | 4 | 58 | med |
| 50 | 0 | 0 | 6 | 1 | 18 | 54 | low |
| 78 | 1 | 0 | 22 | 3 | 5 | 22 | low |
| 93 | 0 | 0 | 21 | 1 | 5 | 41 | low |
| 62 | 0 | 0 | 17 | 1 | 1 | 64 | med |
| 64 | 1 | 0 | 13 | 2 | 3 | 54 | low |
| 78 | 0 | 0 | 18 | 3 | 4 | 39 | low |
| 72 | 0 | 0 | 17 | 2 | 4 | 45 | low |
| 37 | 0 | 0 | 8 | 1 | 0 | ★ | |

# FRUIT

| FOOD | SERVING SIZE | HOUSEHOLD MEASURE |
|---|---|---|
| Figs, dried, tenderized | 1 oz | 1½ figs |
| Fruit and nut mix | 1¼ oz | ¼ cup |
| Fruit cocktail, canned | 5 oz | ½ cup |
| Fruit salad, canned in fruit juice | 4½ oz | ½ cup |
| Grapefruit | 11 oz | 1 large |
| Grapefruit, ruby red segments in juice | 4½ oz | ½ cup |
| Grapes | 3½ oz | 25 grapes (1 small bunch) |
| Kiwi | 6¾ oz | 2 small |
| Kumquats | ¾ oz | 1 average |
| Lemon | ½ oz | 1 wedge |
| Lime | ½ oz | 1 wedge |
| Loganberries | 2½ oz | ½ cup |
| Lychees, canned, in syrup, drained | 3 oz | 7 average |
| Lychees, fresh, B3 variety | 2 oz | 5 lychees |
| Mandarin segments in juice | 4½ oz | ½ cup |
| Mango | 3½ oz | ½ average |
| Mixed fruit, dried | 1 oz | 2 tbsp |
| Mixed nuts and raisins | 1 oz | ¼ cup |
| Mulberries | 2½ oz | ½ cup |
| Nectarine, fresh | 4 oz | 1 average |
| Orange | 7 oz | 1 large |
| Orange & grapefruit segments in juice | 4½ oz | ½ cup |

@ part of GI symbol program     ★ little or no carbs

| CALORIES | FAT (g) | SATURATED FAT (g) | CARBO-HYDRATE (g) | FIBER (g) | SODIUM (mg) | GI | LOW MED HIGH |
|---|---|---|---|---|---|---|---|
| 78 | 0 | 0 | 16 | 4 | 12 | 61 | med |
| 158 | 8 | 2 | 17 | 3 | 19 | 15 | low |
| 68 | 0 | 0 | 16 | 2 | 5 | 55 | low |
| 69 | 0 | 0 | 15 | 2 | 6 | 54 | low |
| 86 | 1 | 0 | 15 | 2 | 12 | 25 | low |
| 77 | 0 | 0 | 20 | 1 | 4 | 47 | low |
| 63 | 0 | 0 | 15 | 1 | 6 | 53 | low |
| 108 | 0 | 0 | 19 | 8 | 11 | 53 | low |
| 13 | 0 | 0 | 2 | 1 | 1 | ★ | |
| 2 | 0 | 0 | 0 | 0 | 0 | ★ | |
| 3 | 0 | 0 | 0 | 0 | 0 | ★ | |
| 51 | 0 | 0 | 4 | 6 | 1 | ★ | |
| 65 | 0 | 0 | 15 | 1 | 5 | 79 | high |
| 32 | 0 | 0 | 7 | 1 | 0 | 57 | med |
| 49 | 0 | 0 | 12 | 1 | 7 | 47 | low |
| 60 | 0 | 0 | 13 | 2 | 1 | 51 | low |
| 78 | 0 | 0 | 18 | 2 | 22 | 60 | med |
| 158 | 8 | 2 | 17 | 3 | 19 | 21 | low |
| 23 | 0 | 0 | 3 | 2 | 4 | ★ | |
| 50 | 0 | 0 | 10 | 2 | 0 | 43 | low |
| 78 | 0 | 0 | 15 | 4 | 4 | 42 | low |
| 74 | 0 | 0 | 19 | 1 | 12 | 53 | low |

# FRUIT

| FOOD | SERVING SIZE | HOUSEHOLD MEASURE |
|------|--------------|-------------------|
| Papaya | 5 oz | 1 small |
| Peach | 7 oz | 2 small |
| Peach and pineapple in fruit juice | 4½ oz | ½ cup |
| Peaches, canned, in heavy syrup | 5 oz | ½ cup |
| Peaches, canned, in light syrup | 4½ oz | ½ cup |
| Peaches, canned, in natural juice | 5½ oz | ¾ cup |
| Peaches, dried | 1 oz | 3 halves |
| Peaches and grapes, canned in fruit juice | 4½ oz | ½ cup |
| Pear | 4 oz | 1 small |
| Pear, canned, in fruit juice | 4½ oz | ½ cup |
| Pear, canned, in natural juice | 5 oz | ¾ pear |
| Pear, dried | 1 oz | 1 ½ halves |
| Pear halves, canned, in reduced-sugar syrup, lite | 3½ oz | ½ pear |
| Pineapple | 6 oz | 1 large slice |
| Pineapple & papaya pieces, canned in juice | 4½ oz | ½ cup |
| Pineapple pieces, canned in fruit juice | 4½ oz | ½ cup |
| Plum | 9 oz | 2 large |
| Prunes, pitted, Sunsweet | 1½ oz | 5 prunes |
| Raisins | ¾ oz | 6 tsp |
| Raspberries | 2 oz | ½ cup |
| Rhubarb, stewed, unsweetened | 3½ oz | ⅓ cup |

@ part of GI symbol program   ★ little or no carbs

| CALORIES | FAT (g) | SATURATED FAT (g) | CARBO-HYDRATE (g) | FIBER (g) | SODIUM (mg) | GI | LOW MED HIGH |
|---|---|---|---|---|---|---|---|
| 59 | 0 | 0 | 12 | 3 | 5 | 56 | med |
| 69 | 0 | 0 | 13 | 3 | 4 | 42 | low |
| 59 | 0 | 0 | 13 | 2 | 6 | 45 | low |
| 66 | 0 | 0 | 14 | 2 | 7 | 58 | med |
| 73 | 0 | 0 | 17 | 2 | 4 | 57 | med |
| 69 | 0 | 0 | 15 | 2 | 8 | 45 | low |
| 80 | 0 | 0 | 16 | 3 | 5 | 35 | low |
| 55 | 0 | 0 | 13 | 2 | 5 | 46 | low |
| 68 | 0 | 0 | 16 | 3 | 2 | 38 | low |
| 62 | 0 | 0 | 14 | 2 | 5 | 43 | low |
| 65 | 0 | 0 | 15 | 2 | 7 | 44 | low |
| 68 | 0 | 0 | 16 | 3 | 3 | 43 | low |
| 62 | 0 | 0 | 15 | 2 | 2 | 25 | low |
| 69 | 2 | 0 | 13 | 4 | 3 | 59 | med |
| 68 | 0 | 0 | 18 | 2 | 6 | 48 | low |
| 74 | 0 | 0 | 19 | 2 | 15 | 49 | low |
| 103 | 0 | 0 | 19 | 6 | 5 | 39 | low |
| 97 | 0 | 0 | 22 | 3 | 38 | 40 | low |
| 60 | 0 | 0 | 14 | 1 | 12 | 64 | med |
| 29 | 0 | 0 | 3 | 3 | 1 | ★ | |
| 19 | 0 | 0 | 1 | 3 | 9 | ★ | |

# FRUIT

| FOOD | SERVING SIZE | HOUSEHOLD MEASURE |
|------|--------------|-------------------|
| Strawberries | 17 oz | 3 cups |
| Tropical fruit and nut mix | 1 oz | 3 tbsp |
| Watermelon | 10 oz | 1 large slice |

@ part of GI symbol program     ★ little or no carbs

| CALORIES | FAT (g) | SATURATED FAT (g) | CARBO-HYDRATE (g) | FIBER (g) | SODIUM (mg) | GI | LOW MED HIGH |
|---|---|---|---|---|---|---|---|
| 115 | 1 | 0 | 13 | 11 | 29 | 40 | low |
| 120 | 4 | 1 | 17 | 1 | 14 | 49 | low |
| 69 | 1 | 0 | 14 | 2 | 6 | 76 | high |

# GLUTEN-FREE PRODUCTS

| FOOD | SERVING SIZE | HOUSEHOLD MEASURE |
|---|---|---|
| Apricot and Apple Fruit Strips | ¾ oz | I strip |
| Apricot spread, no added sugar | I oz | I tbsp |
| Breakfast cereal, Vita-Pro® | I oz | ⅔ cup |
| Buckwheat pancakes, gluten-free, packet mix | ¾ oz | I small |
| Cookie, chocolate-coated | I½ oz | 2 cookies |
| Corn pasta | 2 oz | ½ cup |
| Corn Thins, puffed corn cakes, gluten-free | ¾ oz | 4 slices |
| Marmalade spread, no added sugar | I oz | I tbsp |
| Muesli (Gluten and Wheat free with Psyllium) | I½ oz | ½ cup |
| Muesli Breakfast Bar, gluten-free | ¾ oz | ½ bar |
| Multigrain bread | I oz | I slice |
| Omega Bar (Gluten, Wheat and Dairy free) | I¼ oz | I bar |
| Pancakes, gluten-free, made from packet mix | 3 oz | 2 pancakes |
| Pasta, rice and corn, dry | I oz | ⅙ cup |
| Peach and Pear Fruit Strips | ¾ oz | I strip |
| Plum and Apple Fruit Strips | I oz | I½ strips |
| Raspberry spread, no added sugar | I oz | I tbsp |
| Rice pasta, enriched (Gluten, Maize, Wheat and Soya free), Freedom Foods | ¾ oz | ⅙ cup |

@ part of GI symbol program    ★ little or no carbs

| CALORIES | FAT (g) | SATURATED FAT (g) | CARBO-HYDRATE (g) | FIBER (g) | SODIUM (mg) | GI | LOW MED HIGH |
|---|---|---|---|---|---|---|---|
| 71 | 0 | 0 | 16 | 2 | 5 | 29 | low |
| 56 | 0 | 0 | 13 | 0 | 3 | 29 | low |
| 104 | 1 | 0 | 14 | 6 | 88 | 52 | low |
| 67 | 0 | 0 | 15 | 1 | 95 | 102 | high |
| 183 | 11 | 6 | 18 | 3 | 52 | 35 | low |
| 78 | 1 | 0 | 15 | 3 | 0 | 78 | high |
| 89 | 1 | 0 | 16 | 2 | 60 | 87 | high |
| 61 | 0 | 0 | 14 | 0 | 3 | 27 | low |
| 183 | 11 | 5 | 13 | 7 | 12 | 50 | low |
| 97 | 4 | 2 | 13 | 2 | 6 | 50 | low |
| 91 | 2 | 1 | 15 | 2 | 83 | 79 | high |
| 174 | 4 | 2 | 15 | 3 | 4 | 21 | low |
| 240 | 2 | 0 | 53 | 6 | 640 | 61 | med |
| 79 | 0 | 0 | 19 | 1 | 2 | 76 | high |
| 71 | 0 | 0 | 15 | 3 | 14 | 29 | low |
| 77 | 0 | 0 | 16 | 4 | 10 | 29 | low |
| 60 | 0 | 0 | 14 | 0 | 17 | 26 | low |
| 80 | 0 | 0 | 18 | 1 | 3 | 51 | low |

# GLUTEN-FREE PRODUCTS

| FOOD | SERVING SIZE | HOUSEHOLD MEASURE |
|------|------|------|
| Spaghetti, Enriched (Gluten, Wheat and Soya free), Freedom Foods | ¾ oz | ⅙ cup |
| Spaghetti, rice and split pea, canned in tomato sauce | 4 oz | ½ can |
| Strawberry spread, no added sugar | 1 oz | 1 tbsp |

@ part of GI symbol program    ★ little or no carbs

| CALORIES | FAT (g) | SATURATED FAT (g) | CARBO-HYDRATE (g) | FIBER (g) | SODIUM (mg) | GI | LOW MED HIGH |
|---|---|---|---|---|---|---|---|
| 79 | 0 | 0 | 19 | 1 | 3 | 51 | low |
| 69 | 0 | 0 | 14 | 1 | 440 | 68 | med |
| 60 | 0 | 0 | 14 | 0 | 3 | 29 | low |

# MEALS, PREPARED & CONVENIENCE

| FOOD | SERVING SIZE | HOUSEHOLD MEASURE |
|------|------|------|
| Baked potato with baked beans | 7 oz | 1 medium potato |
| Beef and ale casserole, prepared convenience meal | 10½ oz | 1 meal |
| Burrito, made with corn tortilla, refried beans and tomato salsa | 3½ oz | 1 small burrito |
| Cannelloni, spinach and ricotta, prepared convenience meal | 8 oz | 1 serving |
| Chicken curry and rice, prepared convenience meal | 10 ½ oz | 1 meal |
| Chicken fajitas | 3 oz | 1 fajita |
| Chicken nuggets, frozen, reheated in microwave 5 mins | 4 oz | 6 nuggets |
| Chicken tandoori curry with rice, prepared meal | 10 oz | 1 meal |
| Chow mein, chicken, prepared convenience meal | 10½ | 1 meal |
| Creamy carbonara wholegrain pasta & sauce meal | 5 oz | 1 serving |
| Fish fingers | 2½ oz | 3 fingers |
| French fries, frozen, reheated in microwave | 5 oz | 10 fries |
| French-style chicken with rice, prepared convenience meal | 7 oz | 1 serving |
| Grape leaves, stuffed with rice and lamb, served with tomato sauce | 4 oz | 4 stuffed leaves |

@ part of GI symbol program    ★ little or no carbs

| CALORIES | FAT (g) | SATURATED FAT (g) | CARBO-HYDRATE (g) | FIBER (g) | SODIUM (mg) | GI | LOW MED HIGH |
|---|---|---|---|---|---|---|---|
| 47 | 1 | 0 | 26 | 6 | 251 | 62 | low |
| 444 | 23 | 10 | 17 | 3 | 657 | 53 | low |
| 264 | 13 | 6 | 19 | 2 | 688 | 39 | low |
| 196 | 4 | 2 | 30 | 4 | 573 | 15 | low |
| 640 | 48 | 26 | 20 | 3 | 198 | 45 | low |
| 138 | 8 | 3.8 | 6 | 2 | 175 | 42 | low |
| 288 | 17 | 7 | 16 | 1 | 454 | 46 | low |
| 488 | 22 | 12 | 53 | 2 | 455 | 45 | low |
| 448 | 33 | 12 | 18 | 8 | 990 | 51 | low |
| 148 | 5 | 2 | 21 | 2 | 290 | 39 | low |
| 156 | 8 | 2 | 13 | 1 | 220 | 38 | low |
| 120 | 3 | 0 | 19 | 2 | 25 | 75 | high |
| 287 | 11 | 3 | 32 | 2 | 394 | 36 | low |
| 124 | 4 | 2 | 15 | 2 | 268 | 30 | low |

# MEALS, PREPARED & CONVENIENCE

| FOOD | SERVING SIZE | HOUSEHOLD MEASURE |
|------|------|------|
| Hamburger, commercially prepared | 3 oz | 1 small burger |
| Lamb moussaka, prepared convenience meal | 10½ oz | 1 meal |
| Lasagna, beef, commercially made | 5 oz | 1 serving |
| ⓖ Lean Cuisine®, Burmese Vegetable Curry and Rice | 3½ oz | ⅓ meal |
| ⓖ Lean Cuisine®, Chicken Pomodoro | 5 oz | ½ meal |
| ⓖ Lean Cuisine®, Honey Soy Beef | 5 oz | ½ meal |
| Mashed potato, instant | 4 oz | ½ cup |
| McDonald's Chicken McNuggets® consumed with Sweet 'N Sour Sauce | 4½ oz | 6 nuggets & sauce |
| McDonald's Fillet-O-Fish® Burger | 4½ oz | 1 burger |
| McDonald's Hamburger | 3½ oz | 1 small burger |
| McDonald's McChicken® Burger | 6½ oz | 1 burger |
| NutriSystem, Beef Stroganoff with Noodles | 9 oz | 1 container |
| NutriSystem, Cheese Tortellini | 8 oz | 1 container |
| NutriSystem, Chicken Cacciatore Parmesan | 8 oz | 1 container |
| NutriSystem, Chicken Pasta | 9 oz | 1 container |
| NutriSystem, Hearty Beef Stew | 8 oz | 1 container |
| NutriSystem, Lasagna with Meat Sauce | 8 oz | 1 container |

ⓖ part of GI symbol program     ★ little or no carbs

| CALORIES | FAT (g) | SATURATED FAT (g) | CARBO-HYDRATE (g) | FIBER (g) | SODIUM (mg) | GI | LOW MED HIGH |
|---|---|---|---|---|---|---|---|
| 254 | 10 | 3 | 28 | 1 | 378 | 66 | med |
| 312 | 19 | 4 | 20 | 6 | 620 | 35 | low |
| 190 | 8 | 4 | 17 | 4 | 330 | 47 | low |
| 94 | 3 | 0 | 14 | 2 | 185 | 50 | low |
| 134 | 3 | 0 | 18 | 2 | 308 | 47 | low |
| 133 | 3 | 0 | 20 | 1 | 511 | 47 | low |
| 74 | 0 | 0 | 14 | 2 | 4 | 85 | high |
| 333 | 18 | 3 | 26 | 1 | 627 | 55 | low |
| 310 | 14 | 3 | 30 | 2 | 634 | 66 | med |
| 237 | 9 | 4 | 25 | 2 | 433 | 66 | med |
| 418 | 19 | 3 | 40 | 2 | 706 | 66 | med |
| 240 | 8 | 4 | 21 | 2 | 610 | 41 | low |
| 170 | 2 | 1 | 25 | 2 | 550 | 41 | low |
| 130 | 2 | 1 | 17 | 2 | 560 | 27 | low |
| 180 | 3 | 1 | 23 | 3 | 610 | 41 | low |
| 180 | 4 | 2 | 15 | 2 | 490 | 26 | low |
| 260 | 8 | 4 | 26 | 6 | 730 | 26 | low |

# MEALS, PREPARED & CONVENIENCE

| FOOD | SERVING SIZE | HOUSEHOLD MEASURE |
|------|------|------|
| NutriSystem, Pot Roast | 10 oz | 1 container |
| NutriSystem, Rotini with Meatballs | 9 oz | 1 container |
| NutriSystem, Thin Crust Pizza with Cheese | 3 oz | 1 container |
| NutriSystem, Whipped Sweet Potatoes | 2 oz | 1 container |
| Pizza, cheese | 5 oz | 2 slices |
| Pizza, Super Supreme, pan, Pizza Hut | 1¾ oz | 1/16 of large pizza |
| Pizza, Super Supreme, Thin 'n Crispy, Pizza Hut | 2½ oz | 1/8 of large pizza |
| Pizza, Veggie Lovers®, Thin 'n Crispy, Pizza Hut | 1¾ oz | 1/16 of large pizza |
| President's Choice® Blue Menu™ 3-Rice Bayou Blend Rice & Beans Sidedish | 2 oz | ¼ package |
| President's Choice® Blue Menu™ 9-Vegetable Vegetarian Patty (frozen) | 4 oz | 1 patty |
| President's Choice® Blue Menu™ 4-Rice Pilaf Rice & Beans Sidedish | 2 oz | ¼ package |
| President's Choice® Blue Menu™ Barley Risotto with Herbed Chicken | 10 oz | 1 container |

@ part of GI symbol program ★ little or no carbs

| CALORIES | FAT (g) | SATURATED FAT (g) | CARBO-HYDRATE (g) | FIBER (g) | SODIUM (mg) | GI | LOW MED HIGH |
|---|---|---|---|---|---|---|---|
| 270 | 7 | 2 | 16 | 2 | 780 | 31 | low |
| 250 | 9 | 4 | 25 | 4 | 770 | 29 | low |
| 220 | 10 | 6 | 23 | 1 | 760 | 36 | low |
| 200 | 5 | 3 | 24 | 5 | 630 | 36 | low |
| 429 | 18 | 6 | 52 | 3 | 266 | 60 | med |
| 127 | 5 | 2 | 14 | 1 | 241 | 36 | low |
| 197 | 8 | 4 | 18 | 2 | 566 | 30 | low |
| 123 | 4 | 2 | 15 | 1 | 284 | 49 | low |
| 180 | 1 | 0 | 34 | 3 | 360 | 44 | low |
| 160 | 2 | 0 | 29 | 4 | 540 | 54 | low |
| 170 | 0 | 0 | 36 | 2 | 330 | 46 | low |
| 290 | 6 | 2 | 37 | 5 | 800 | 38 | low |

# MEALS, PREPARED & CONVENIENCE

| FOOD | SERVING SIZE | HOUSEHOLD MEASURE |
|------|------|------|
| President's Choice® Blue Menu™ Cauliflower Topped Shepherd's Pie | 8 oz | ¼ pie |
| President's Choice® Blue Menu™ Chicken Curry with Vegetables | 10 oz | I container |
| President's Choice® Blue Menu™ Deluxe Cheddar Macaroni & Cheese Dinner | 2 oz | ⅓ packet |
| President's Choice® Blue Menu™ Ginger Glazed Salmon | II oz | I container |
| President's Choice® Blue Menu™ Lentil and Bean Vegetarian Patty | 4 oz | I patty |
| President's Choice® Blue Menu™ Linguine with Shrimp Marinara | II oz | I container |
| President's Choice® Blue Menu™ Medagiloni with Ricotta & Sun-Dried Tomatoes | 4 oz | ¾ cup |
| President's Choice® Blue Menu™ Pasta Sauce, Tomato and Basil | 4 oz | ½ cup |
| President's Choice® Blue Menu™ Penne with Roasted Vegetable Entrée | II oz | I container |
| President's Choice® Blue Menu™ Rotini with Chicken Pesto (entrée) | 10 oz | I meal |
| President's Choice® Blue Menu™ Rice & Lentils Espana Sidedish | 2 oz | ¼ package |

@ part of GI symbol program     ★ little or no carbs

| CALORIES | FAT (g) | SATURATED FAT (g) | CARBO-HYDRATE (g) | FIBER (g) | SODIUM (mg) | GI | LOW MED HIGH |
|---|---|---|---|---|---|---|---|
| 220 | 9 | 5 | 13 | 1 | 590 | 21 | low |
| 190 | 5 | 1 | 11 | 6 | 560 | 26 | low |
| 230 | 3 | 2 | 39 | 3 | 450 | 34 | low |
| 300 | 4 | 1 | 45 | 5 | 570 | 40 | low |
| 170 | 2 | 0 | 27 | 4 | 490 | 55 | low |
| 240 | 4 | 1 | 28 | 8 | 750 | 40 | low |
| 290 | 5 | 3 | 47 | 6 | 300 | 54 | low |
| 70 | 2 | 0 | 8 | 2 | 480 | 33 | low |
| 320 | 6 | 3 | 43 | 9 | 750 | 39 | low |
| 370 | 8 | 2 | 44 | 6 | 670 | 57 | med |
| 180 | 1 | 0 | 38 | 2 | 350 | 49 | low |

# MEALS, PREPARED & CONVENIENCE

| FOOD | SERVING SIZE | HOUSEHOLD MEASURE |
|---|---|---|
| President's Choice® Blue Menu™ Sesame Ginger Chicken with Vegetables (entrée) | 10 oz | 1 meal |
| President's Choice® Blue Menu™ Stone Baked Whole Wheat Pizza - Vegetable, Pesto & Feta Cheese | 5 oz | ½ pizza |
| President's Choice® Blue Menu™ Tomato & Herb Chicken w/ Vegetables Entrée | 10 oz | 1 tray |
| President's Choice® Blue Menu™ Tricolour Linguini Sun-Dried Tomato, Basil and Original Nest | 4 oz | ⅓ package |
| President's Choice® Blue Menu™ Vegetarian Chili | 8 oz | 1 cup |
| President's Choice® Blue Menu™ Whole Grain Pizza Kit | 3¼ oz | ½ pizza |
| President's Choice® Blue Menu™ Yellow Curry Chicken (entrée) | 10 oz | 1 meal |
| Sausages | 4 oz | 2 sausages |
| Sausages and mash potato, prepared convenience meal | 10 oz | 1 meal |
| Shepherds' pie | 10½ oz | 1 meal |
| Sirloin steak with mixed vegetables and mashed potato, homemade | 10½ oz | 1 meal |
| Spaghetti bolognese, homemade | 10½ oz | 1 meal |

@ part of GI symbol program     ★ little or no carbs

| CALORIES | FAT (g) | SATURATED FAT (g) | CARBO-HYDRATE (g) | FIBER (g) | SODIUM (mg) | GI | LOW MED HIGH |
|---|---|---|---|---|---|---|---|
| 190 | 5 | 1 | 17 | 1 | 750 | 44 | low |
| 240 | 7 | 2 | 28 | 5 | 650 | 54 | low |
| 150 | 4 | 1 | 14 | 3 | 590 | 29 | low |
| 350 | 5 | 1 | 61 | 4 | 45 | 42 | low |
| 200 | 3 | 1 | 34 | 5 | 480 | 39 | low |
| 190 | 3 | 1 | 33 | 5 | 450 | 59 | med |
| 200 | 7 | 6 | 14 | 3 | 810 | 25 | low |
| 303 | 21 | 10 | 9 | 3 | 1079 | 28 | low |
| 256 | 13 | 6 | 27 | 6 | 1305 | 61 | med |
| 320 | 16 | 7 | 22 | 3 | 1275 | 66 | med |
| 309 | 13 | 5 | 25 | 6 | 122 | 66 | med |
| 468 | 11 | 4 | 65 | 5 | 420 | 52 | low |

# MEALS, PREPARED & CONVENIENCE

| FOOD | SERVING SIZE | HOUSEHOLD MEASURE |
|------|------|------|
| Stirfried vegetables with chicken and boiled white rice, homemade | 10½ oz | 1 meal |
| Sushi, salmon | 2¾ oz | 3 pieces |
| Taco shells, cornmeal-based, baked | 1 oz | 2 regular size |

@ part of GI symbol program   ★ little or no carbs

| CALORIES | FAT (g) | SATURATED FAT (g) | CARBO-HYDRATE (g) | FIBER (g) | SODIUM (mg) | GI | LOW MED HIGH |
|---|---|---|---|---|---|---|---|
| 344 | 4 | 1 | 62 | 5 | 319 | 73 | high |
| | | | | | | | |
| 102 | 1 | 0 | 19 | 1 | 291 | 48 | low |
| 120 | 6 | 1 | 16 | 2 | 95 | 68 | med |

# MEAT, SEAFOOD, EGGS & PROTEIN

| FOOD | SERVING SIZE | HOUSEHOLD MEASURE |
|------|------|------|
| Bacon, fried | 1 oz | 1 small slice |
| Bacon, grilled | 1 oz | 1 slice |
| Beef, corned silverside | ¾ oz | 1 slice |
| Beef, corned silverside, canned | 1¾ oz | 2 slices |
| Beef, roast | 1 oz | 2 slices |
| Beef steak, fat trimmed | 6 oz | 1 medium |
| Brains, cooked | 2 oz | ½ cup |
| Burger, fried | 1¾ oz | 1 average |
| Calamari, fried | 2 oz | ½ cup |
| Calamari rings, squid, not battered or crumbed | 3 oz | 5 rings |
| Chicken breast, baked without skin | 3 oz | ⅓ small |
| Chicken breast, grilled without skin | 3 oz | ⅓ small |
| Chicken chopped, cooked | 3½ oz | ½ cup |
| Chicken drumstick, grilled without skin | 1½ oz | 1 small |
| Chicken loaf | ¾ oz | 1 slice |
| Chicken roll | ¾ oz | 1 slice |
| Chicken thigh fillet grilled, without skin | 1¾ oz | ½ large |
| Chicken wing grilled, without skin | ¾ oz | 1 medium |
| Cod, fried | 4 oz | 1 fillet |

@ part of GI symbol program   ★ little or no carbs

| CALORIES | FAT (g) | SATURATED FAT (g) | CARBO-HYDRATE (g) | FIBER (g) | SODIUM (mg) | GI | LOW MED HIGH |
|---|---|---|---|---|---|---|---|
| 38 | 2 | 1 | 1 | 0 | 500 | ★ | |
| 49 | 2 | 1 | 1 | 0 | 735 | ★ | |
| 23 | 1 | 1 | 0 | 0 | 213 | ★ | |
| 96 | 6 | 2 | 0 | 0 | 570 | ★ | |
| 44 | 1 | 1 | 0 | 0 | 17 | ★ | |
| 356 | 17 | 7 | 0 | 0 | 119 | ★ | |
| 89 | 6 | 2 | 0 | 0 | 73 | ★ | |
| 101 | 6 | 1 | 3 | 0 | 241 | ★ | |
| 70 | 3 | 1 | 0 | 0 | 192 | ★ | |
| 78 | 1 | 0 | 2 | 0 | 37 | ★ | |
| 140 | 6 | 2 | 0 | 0 | 65 | ★ | |
| 150 | 7 | 2 | 0 | 0 | 70 | ★ | |
| 204 | 11 | 3 | 0 | 0 | 101 | ★ | |
| 78 | 3 | 1 | 0 | 0 | 50 | ★ | |
| 42 | 2 | 1 | 2 | 0 | 172 | ★ | |
| 31 | 2 | 1 | 1 | 0 | 142 | ★ | |
| 113 | 7 | 2 | 0 | 0 | 55 | ★ | |
| 37 | 2 | 1 | 0 | 0 | 19 | ★ | |
| 192 | 10 | 3 | 3 | 1 | 163 | ★ | |

# MEAT, SEAFOOD, EGGS & PROTEIN

| FOOD | SERVING SIZE | HOUSEHOLD MEASURE |
|------|------|------|
| Crab, cooked | 2 oz | ½ cup |
| Dory, fried | 4 oz | 1 fillet |
| Duck, roasted, without skin | 2 oz | ½ breast |
| Egg, whole, raw | 2 fl oz | 1 average |
| Egg white, raw | 1 fl oz | 1 average |
| Egg yolk, raw | ½ fl oz | 1 average |
| Flounder, fried | 4 oz | 1 fillet |
| Frankfurter | 2 oz | 1 average |
| Ham, canned leg | 1½ oz | 1 thick slice |
| Hamburger pattie | 2¾ oz | 1 pattie |
| Kingfish (Mackerel), fried | 4 oz | 1 fillet |
| Lamb, ground, cooked | 3½ oz | ½ cup |
| Lamb, grilled chop, fat trimmed | 1¾ oz | 1 medium |
| Lamb, roasted loin, fat trimmed | 2 oz | 1 thick slice |
| Ling (Lingcod), fried | 4 oz | 1 fillet |
| Liver, cooked | 2 oz | ½ cup |
| Liverwurst | 1 oz | 2 slices |
| Lobster, cooked | 2 oz | ½ cup |
| Mullet, fried | 4 oz | 1 fillet |
| Mussels, cooked | 2 oz | ½ cup |
| Nutolene | 3 oz | 2 thick slices |
| Ocean perch, fried | 4 oz | 1 fillet |
| Octopus, cooked | 2 oz | ½ cup |

@ part of GI symbol program      ★ little or no carbs

| CALORIES | FAT (g) | SATURATED FAT (g) | CARBO-HYDRATE (g) | FIBER (g) | SODIUM (mg) | GI | LOW MED HIGH |
|---|---|---|---|---|---|---|---|
| 68 | 0 | 0 | 1 | 0 | 218 | ★ | |
| 203 | 10 | 3 | 3 | 1 | 181 | ★ | |
| 156 | 8 | 2 | 0 | 0 | 81 | ★ | |
| 77 | 6 | 2 | 0 | 0 | 72 | ★ | |
| 15 | 0 | 0 | 0 | 0 | 54 | ★ | |
| 53 | 5 | 2 | 0 | 0 | 10 | ★ | |
| 201 | 10 | 3 | 3 | 1 | 148 | ★ | |
| 144 | 11 | 4 | 1 | 0 | 139 | ★ | |
| 45 | 2 | 1 | 0 | 0 | 500 | ★ | |
| 197 | 14 | 6 | 0 | 0 | 52 | ★ | |
| 261 | 13 | 4 | 4 | 1 | 136 | ★ | |
| 218 | 13 | 7 | 0 | 0 | 80 | ★ | |
| 108 | 5 | 3 | 0 | 0 | 36 | ★ | |
| 141 | 10 | 5 | 0 | 0 | 34 | ★ | |
| 204 | 10 | 3 | 3 | 1 | 230 | ★ | |
| 158 | 8 | 3 | 2 | 0 | 53 | ★ | |
| 92 | 8 | 3 | 0 | 0 | 244 | ★ | |
| 53 | 1 | 0 | 0 | 0 | 213 | ★ | |
| 281 | 17 | 6 | 4 | 1 | 234 | ★ | |
| 76 | 2 | 1 | 4 | 1 | 562 | ★ | |
| 214 | 18 | 3 | 4 | 2 | 281 | ★ | |
| 210 | 10 | 3 | 4 | 1 | 147 | ★ | |
| 69 | 1 | 0 | 1 | 0 | 204 | ★ | |

# MEAT, SEAFOOD, EGGS & PROTEIN

| FOOD | SERVING SIZE | HOUSEHOLD MEASURE |
|---|---|---|
| Oysters, natural, plain | 3 oz | 6 medium |
| Pancetta | ¾ oz | 1 slice |
| Pepperoni | ¾ oz | 1 slice |
| Pork, grilled chops, fat trimmed | 3 oz | 1 medium |
| Prosciutto | 1½ oz | 1 slice |
| Quail | 2¾ oz | 1 average |
| Salami | ¾ oz | 1 slice |
| Salmon, pink, no added salt, drained | 2 oz | ⅔ small can |
| Salmon, red, no added salt, drained | 2 oz | ⅔ small can |
| Sardines, canned in oil, drained | 2 oz | ⅔ small can |
| Sausages, fried | 2 oz | 1 sausage |
| Scallops, cooked | 2 oz | ½ cup |
| Seafood marinara, canned | 2 oz | ⅔ small can |
| Shark, fried | 4 oz | 1 fillet |
| Shrimp | 1 oz | 4 large shrimp |
| Shrimp, cooked | 2 oz | ½ cup |
| Snapper, fried | 4 oz | 1 fillet |
| Sole, fried | 4 oz | 1 fillet |
| Spam, lite | 2 oz | 2 slices |
| Spam, regular | 1½ oz | 2 slices |
| Speck | 3½ oz | 1 slice |
| Steak, lean | 7 oz | 1 medium steak |

© part of GI symbol program    ★ little or no carbs

| CALORIES | FAT (g) | SATURATED FAT (g) | CARBO-HYDRATE (g) | FIBER (g) | SODIUM (mg) | GI | LOW MED HIGH |
|---|---|---|---|---|---|---|---|
| 57 | 2 | 1 | 3 | 0 | 177 | ★ | |
| 40 | 3 | 1 | 0 | 0 | 275 | ★ | |
| 106 | 9 | 4 | 1 | 0 | 365 | ★ | |
| 171 | 7 | 3 | 0 | 0 | 71 | ★ | |
| 51 | 2 | 1 | 0 | 0 | 753 | ★ | |
| 151 | 7 | 2 | 0 | 0 | 45 | ★ | |
| 98 | 9 | 3 | 0 | 0 | 336 | ★ | |
| 90 | 4 | 1 | 0 | 0 | 67 | ★ | |
| 119 | 7 | 2 | 0 | 0 | 67 | ★ | |
| 137 | 10 | 3 | 0 | 0 | 372 | ★ | |
| 239 | 17 | 8 | 4 | 2 | 928 | 28 | low |
| 56 | 1 | 0 | 0 | 0 | 91 | ★ | |
| 67 | 1 | 0 | 3 | 1 | 367 | ★ | |
| 231 | 9 | 2 | 3 | 1 | 164 | ★ | |
| 28 | 0 | 0 | 0 | 0 | 63 | ★ | |
| 55 | 1 | 0 | 0 | 0 | 228 | ★ | |
| 251 | 12 | 4 | 4 | 1 | 181 | ★ | |
| 206 | 11 | 3 | 3 | 1 | 186 | ★ | |
| 96 | 8 | 3 | 2 | 0 | 580 | ★ | |
| 133 | 12 | 5 | 1 | 0 | 628 | ★ | |
| 212 | 14 | 5 | 0 | 0 | 1480 | ★ | |
| 238 | 10 | 5 | 0 | 0 | 72 | ★ | |

# MEAT, SEAFOOD, EGGS & PROTEIN

| FOOD | SERVING SIZE | HOUSEHOLD MEASURE |
|------|------|------|
| Tofu, plain, unsweetened | 3½ oz | I serve |
| Tofu, cooked | 4½ oz | ½ cup |
| Trevally, fried | 4 oz | I fillet |
| Trout, cooked | 4 oz | I fillet |
| Trout, fresh or frozen | 5¾ oz | I medium trout |
| Trout, fried | 4 oz | I fillet |
| Tuna, cooked | 4 oz | I fillet |
| Tuna in brine, drained | 2 oz | ⅔ small can |
| Tuna in oil | 2 oz | ⅔ small can |
| Turkey breast, deli-sliced | ¾ oz | I slice |
| Turkey breast, rolled roast | 3 oz | 2 thick slices |
| Turkey breast, smoked, without skin | 3 oz | 2 thick slices |
| Turkey leg, roasted without skin | 3 oz | 2 thick slices |
| Turkey, roasted breast without skin | 2¾ oz | 2 thick slices |
| Veal, roasted, fat trimmed | 3 oz | 2 thick slices |
| Vegetarian sausages | 3 oz | I thick |

@ part of GI symbol program    ★ little or no carbs

| CALORIES | FAT (g) | SATURATED FAT (g) | CARBO-HYDRATE (g) | FIBER (g) | SODIUM (mg) | GI | LOW MED HIGH |
|---|---|---|---|---|---|---|---|
| 127 | 7 | 1 | 0 | 7 | 40 | ★ | |
| 96 | 6 | 1 | 1 | 0 | 5 | ★ | |
| 234 | 12 | 3 | 3 | 1 | 131 | ★ | |
| 164 | 6 | 1 | 0 | 0 | 70 | ★ | |
| 238 | 8 | 2 | 0 | 0 | 104 | ★ | |
| 200 | 9 | 3 | 4 | 1 | 129 | ★ | |
| 213 | 8 | 3 | 0 | 0 | 57 | ★ | |
| 76 | 2 | 1 | 0 | 0 | 253 | ★ | |
| 177 | 14 | 2 | 0 | 0 | 253 | ★ | |
| 34 | 1 | 0 | 0 | 0 | 46 | ★ | |
| 132 | 3 | 1 | 0 | 0 | 179 | ★ | |
| 132 | 3 | 1 | 0 | 0 | 179 | ★ | |
| 146 | 6 | 2 | 0 | 0 | 145 | ★ | |
| 117 | 3 | 1 | 0 | 0 | 158 | ★ | |
| 122 | 1 | 0 | 0 | 0 | 43 | ★ | |
| 109 | 4 | 1 | 3 | 2 | 381 | ★ | |

# NUTRITIONAL SUPPLEMENTS

| FOOD | SERVING SIZE | HOUSEHOLD MEASURE |
|---|---|---|
| Ensure™ bar, chocolate fudge brownie | 1¼ oz | 1 bar |
| Ensure™ Hospital, nutritional supplement powder, prepared with water | 8½ fl oz | 1 cup |
| Ensure Plus™, vanilla | 8 fl oz | 1 can |
| Ensure®, vanilla drink | 3 fl oz | ⅓ cup |
| Ensure®, vanilla drink | 8 floz | 1 can |
| Jevity®, fiber-enriched drink | 8 floz | 1 can |
| Jevity® HiCal, enteral nutritional supplement | 8 floz | 1 can |
| Nutrimeal™ meal replacement drink, Usana | 8 fl oz | 1 cup |
| Promote with Fibre™ nutritional supplement | 8 fl oz | 1 can |
| ProSure™, ready-to-drink nutritional supplement, vanilla flavor | 8 fl oz | 1 can |
| Sustagen® Drink, Dutch Chocolate | 3 fl oz | ⅓ cup |
| Sustagen™, Dutch Chocolate | 8 fl oz | 1 tetra pack |
| Sustagen™ Hospital with extra fiber, drink made from powdered mix | 8½ fl oz | 1 cup |
| TwoCal HN™, high nitrogen nutritional supplement, vanilla flavor | 8 fl oz | 1 can |

ⓖ part of GI symbol program       ★ little or no carbs

| CALORIES | FAT (g) | SATURATED FAT (g) | CARBO-HYDRATE (g) | FIBER (g) | SODIUM (mg) | GI | LOW MED HIGH |
|---|---|---|---|---|---|---|---|
| 140 | 4 | | 20 | 2 | | 43 | low |
| 250 | 8 | | 32 | 2 | 210 | 51 | low |
| 350 | 11 | 1 | 47 | 3 | 220 | 40 | low |
| 101 | 2 | 0 | 16 | 0 | 80 | 48 | low |
| 250 | 6 | 1 | 40 | 0 | 200 | 48 | low |
| 250 | 8 | | 36 | 3 | 220 | 48 | low |
| 355 | 12 | | 46 | 5 | 330 | 59 | med |
| 163 | 5 | 1 | 17 | 6 | 189 | 20 | low |
| 237 | 7 | | 32 | 3 | 310 | 49 | low |
| 300 | 6 | 3 | 42 | 5 | 360 | 55 | low |
| 84 | 1 | 0 | 14 | 0 | 92 | 31 | low |
| 225 | 6 | 1 | 34 | 0 | 186 | 31 | low |
| 320 | 3 | 2 | 44 | 5 | 220 | 33 | low |
| 475 | 22 | | 50 | 1 | 345 | 55 | low |

# NUTS & SEEDS

| FOOD | SERVING SIZE | HOUSEHOLD MEASURE |
|------|------|------|
| Almonds, raw | ½ oz | 1 tbsp |
| Almonds, roasted | ½ oz | 1 tbsp |
| Blue Diamond Whole Natural Almonds | 1 oz | 24 nuts |
| Brazil nuts | ½ oz | 1 tbsp |
| Cashew nuts, raw | ½ oz | 1 tbsp |
| Cashew nuts, roasted and salted | ½ oz | 1 tbsp |
| Coconut, fresh | ½ oz | 1 tbsp |
| Coconut cream | 4 fl oz | ½ cup |
| Coconut milk, canned | 4 fl oz | ½ cup |
| Coconut milk, fresh | 4 fl oz | ½ cup |
| Flaxseeds | ½ oz | 1 tbsp |
| Hazelnuts | ½ oz | 1 tbsp |
| Macadamia nuts, raw | ½ oz | 1 tbsp |
| Macadamia nuts, roasted | ½ oz | 1 tbsp |
| Mixed nuts, fruit, seeds | ½ oz | 1 tbsp |
| Mixed nuts, raw | ½ oz | 1 tbsp |
| Mixed nuts, roasted, salted | ½ oz | 1 tbsp |
| Mixed nuts, roasted, unsalted | ½ oz | 1 tbsp |
| Nut & raisin mix | ½ oz | 1 tbsp |
| Nut & seed mix | ½ oz | 1 tbsp |
| Peanut butter | ½ oz | 3 tsp |
| Peanut butter, no added sugar | ½ oz | 3 tsp |
| Peanuts, raw | 1 oz | 1 tbsp |

@ part of GI symbol program     ★ little or no carbs

| CALORIES | FAT (g) | SATURATED FAT (g) | CARBO-HYDRATE (g) | FIBER (g) | SODIUM (mg) | GI | LOW MED HIGH |
|---|---|---|---|---|---|---|---|
| 79 | 7 | 1 | 1 | 1 | 1 | ★ | |
| 84 | 8 | 1 | 1 | 1 | 1 | ★ | |
| 160 | 14 | 1 | 6 | 3 | 0 | 25 | low |
| 90 | 9 | 2 | 0 | 1 | 0 | ★ | |
| 76 | 6 | 1 | 2 | 1 | 1 | 22 | low |
| 83 | 7 | 1 | 3 | 1 | 38 | 22 | low |
| 37 | 4 | 3 | 1 | 1 | 2 | ★ | |
| 263 | 26 | 23 | 5 | 2 | 27 | ★ | |
| 261 | 26 | 23 | 5 | 2 | 27 | ★ | |
| 302 | 30 | 27 | 4 | 3 | 19 | ★ | |
| 46 | 3 | 0 | 2 | | 7 | ★ | |
| 84 | 8 | 0 | 1 | 1 | 0 | ★ | |
| 96 | 10 | 1 | 1 | 1 | 0 | ★ | |
| 96 | 10 | 1 | 1 | 1 | 72 | ★ | |
| 62 | 4 | 1 | 4 | 1 | 5 | 21 | low |
| 79 | 7 | 1 | 1 | 1 | 0 | ★ | |
| 84 | 7 | 1 | 4 | 1 | 95 | 24 | low |
| 81 | 7 | 1 | 1 | 1 | 0 | ★ | |
| 68 | 5 | 1 | 5 | 1 | 21 | ★ | |
| 81 | 7 | 1 | 1 | 1 | 21 | ★ | |
| 104 | 8 | 1 | 2 | 1 | 51 | ★ | |
| 107 | 9 | 2 | 1 | 2 | 51 | ★ | |
| 155 | 13 | 2 | 3 | 2 | 0 | 23 | low |

# NUTS & SEEDS

| FOOD | SERVING SIZE | HOUSEHOLD MEASURE |
|------|--------------|-------------------|
| Peanuts, roasted | ½ oz | 3 tsp |
| Pecans, raw | ½ oz | 1 tbsp |
| Pine nuts | ½ oz | 1 tbsp |
| Pistachio nuts, raw | ½ oz | 1 tbsp |
| Pistachio nuts, roasted | ½ oz | 1 tbsp |
| Poppy seeds | ¼ oz | 2 tsp |
| Pumpkin seeds, raw | ½ oz | 1 tbsp |
| Sesame seeds | ⅓ oz | 1 tbsp |
| Sunflower seeds, raw | ½ oz | 1 tbsp |
| Sunflower seeds, roasted | ½ oz | 1 tbsp |
| Walnuts | ½ oz | 1 tbsp |

@ part of GI symbol program     ★ little or no carbs

| CALORIES | FAT (g) | SATURATED FAT (g) | CARBO-HYDRATE (g) | FIBER (g) | SODIUM (mg) | GI | LOW MED HIGH |
|---|---|---|---|---|---|---|---|
| 115 | 10 | 1 | 3 | 1 | 61 | 23 | low |
| 93 | 9 | 1 | 2 | 1 | 0 | ★ | |
| 91 | 9 | 1 | 1 | 1 | 0 | ★ | |
| 79 | 7 | 1 | 2 | 1 | 1 | ★ | |
| 77 | 6 | 1 | 2 | 1 | 83 | ★ | |
| 26 | 2 | 0 | 0 | 1 | 1 | ★ | |
| 75 | 6 | 1 | 2 | 1 | 2 | ★ | |
| 52 | 4 | 1 | 1 | 1 | 1 | ★ | |
| 75 | 7 | 1 | 0 | 1 | 0 | ★ | |
| 77 | 7 | 1 | 0 | 1 | 81 | ★ | |
| 90 | 9 | 1 | 0 | 1 | 0 | ★ | |

# OILS & DRESSINGS

| FOOD | SERVING SIZE | HOUSEHOLD MEASURE |
|------|------|------|
| Caesar salad dressing | 1 fl oz | 1½ tbsp |
| Canola oil | ⅓ fl oz | 2 tsp |
| Copha | ⅓ oz | 2 tsp |
| Cream, pure, >35% fat | 1 fl oz | 1½ tbsp |
| Cream, sour, >35% fat | 1 oz | 1½ tbsp |
| Cream, thickened, >35% fat | ¾ fl oz | 1 tbsp |
| Dripping, pork | ⅓ fl oz | 2 tsp |
| French dressing | 1 fl oz | 1½ tbsp |
| French dressing, fat free, artificially sweetened | 1 fl oz | 1½ tbsp |
| Ghee | ⅓ oz | 2 tsp |
| Italian dressing | 1 fl oz | 1½ tbsp |
| Italian dressing, fat free, artificially sweetened | 1 fl oz | 1½ tbsp |
| Lard | ⅓ oz | 2 tsp |
| Margarine, cooking | ⅓ oz | 2 tsp |
| Mayonnaise | ½ fl oz | 1 tbsp |
| Mayonnaise, creamy, 97% fat free | ¾ fl oz | 1 tbsp |
| Salad dressing, homemade oil & vinegar | 1 fl oz | 1½ tbsp |
| Safflower oil | ⅓ fl oz | 2 tsp |
| Sesame oil | ⅓ fl oz | 2 tsp |
| Soybean oil | ⅓ fl oz | 2 tsp |
| Suet | ⅓ oz | 2 tsp |
| Sunflower oil | ⅓ fl oz | 2 tsp |

| CALORIES | FAT (g) | SATURATED FAT (g) | CARBO-HYDRATE (g) | FIBER (g) | SODIUM (mg) | GI | LOW MED HIGH |
|---|---|---|---|---|---|---|---|
| 149 | 17 | 2 | 0 | 0 | 6 | ★ | |
| 89 | 10 | 1 | 0 | 0 | 0 | ★ | |
| 83 | 9 | 9 | 0 | 0 | 0 | ★ | |
| 120 | 13 | 9 | 1 | 0 | 6 | ★ | |
| 120 | 13 | 8 | 1 | 0 | 9 | ★ | |
| 70 | 7 | 5 | 1 | 0 | 10 | ★ | |
| 83 | 9 | 4 | 0 | 0 | 0 | ★ | |
| 82 | 7 | 1 | 4 | 0 | 567 | ★ | |
| 3 | 0 | 0 | 0 | 0 | 514 | ★ | |
| 97 | 11 | 7 | 0 | 0 | 0 | ★ | |
| 95 | 9 | 1 | 2 | 0 | 399 | ★ | |
| 4 | 0 | 0 | 0 | 0 | 239 | ★ | |
| 83 | 9 | 4 | 0 | 0 | 0 | ★ | |
| 72 | 8 | 4 | 0 | 0 | 113 | ★ | |
| 56 | 5 | 1 | 3 | 0 | 122 | ★ | |
| 24 | 1 | 0 | 5 | 0 | 152 | ★ | |
| 178 | 20 | 2 | 0 | 0 | 7 | ★ | |
| 89 | 10 | 1 | 0 | 0 | 0 | ★ | |
| 89 | 10 | 1 | 0 | 0 | 0 | ★ | |
| 89 | 10 | 2 | 0 | 0 | 0 | ★ | |
| 76 | 8 | 5 | 1 | 0 | 0 | ★ | |
| 89 | 10 | 1 | 0 | 0 | 0 | ★ | |

# OILS & DRESSINGS

| FOOD | | SERVING SIZE | HOUSEHOLD MEASURE |
|---|---|---|---|
| Tartar sauce | | 1 fl oz | 1½ tbsp |
| Thousand Island dressing | | ¾ fl oz | 1 tbsp |
| Vinegar | | ½ fl oz | 1 tbsp |

Ⓖ part of GI symbol program    ★ little or no carbs

| CALORIES | FAT (g) | SATURATED FAT (g) | CARBO-HYDRATE (g) | FIBER (g) | SODIUM (mg) | GI | LOW MED HIGH |
|---|---|---|---|---|---|---|---|
| 71 | 7 | 1 | 2 | 0 | 157 | ★ | |
| 56 | 5 | 1 | 4 | 0 | 210 | ★ | |
| 3 | 0 | 0 | 0 | 0 | 1 | ★ | |

# PASTA & NOODLES

| FOOD | SERVING SIZE | HOUSEHOLD MEASURE |
|---|---|---|
| Beef ravioli, fresh, commercially made | 5 oz | 1 serving |
| Beef & vegetable ravioli, fresh, commercially made | 5 oz | 1 serving |
| Meat pasta sauce | 6 oz | 1 serving |
| Cannelloni, spinach and ricotta, prepared convenience meal | 8 oz | 1 serving |
| Capellini pasta, white, boiled | 2 oz | ⅓ cup |
| Cheese & vegetable ravioli, fresh, commercially made | 5 oz | 1 serving |
| Cheese tortellini, cooked | 1¾ oz | ⅓ cup |
| Chicken & garlic ravioli, fresh, commercially made | 5 oz | 1 serving |
| Corn pasta, gluten-free, boiled | 1¾ oz | ⅓ cup |
| Couscous, boiled 5 mins | 5½ oz | 1 cup |
| Creamy carbonara wholegrain pasta & sauce meal | 5 oz | 1 serving |
| Creamy sun-dried tomato pasta sauce | 6 oz | 1 serving |
| Fettuccine, egg, fresh | 5 oz | 1 serving |
| Fusilli twists, tricolor, boiled | 2½ oz | ½ cup |
| Gnocchi, cooked | 1¾ oz | ¼ cup |
| ⓖ Israeli Couscous, Osem brand, boiled | 2.2 oz | ½ cup |
| Italian tomato & garlic pasta sauce | 6 oz | 1 serving |
| Lasagna, beef, commercially made | 5 oz | 1 serving |

ⓖ part of GI symbol program   ★ little or no carbs

| CALORIES | FAT (g) | SATURATED FAT (g) | CARBO-HYDRATE (g) | FIBER (g) | SODIUM (mg) | GI | LOW MED HIGH |
|---|---|---|---|---|---|---|---|
| 279 | 8 | 4 | 40 | 3 | 620 | 43 | low |
| 330 | 9 | 4 | 45 | 5 | 550 | 47 | low |
| 154 | 6 | 2 | 13 | 0 | 743 | 24 | low |
| 196 | 4 | 2 | 30 | 4 | 573 | 15 | low |
| 74 | 0 | 0 | 15 | 1 | 34 | 45 | low |
| 300 | 5 | 2 | 46 | 4 | 649 | 51 | low |
| 98 | 2 | 0 | 15 | 1 | 115 | 50 | low |
| 263 | 6 | 2 | 38 | 3 | 508 | 44 | low |
| 59 | 0 | 0 | 13 | 2 | 0 | 78 | high |
| 73 | 0 | 0 | 15 | 0 | 2 | 65 | med |
| 148 | 5 | 2 | 21 | 2 | 290 | 39 | low |
| 178 | 12 | 8 | 15 | 0 | 354 | 19 | low |
| 204 | 3 | 1 | 36 | 3 | 4 | 54 | low |
| 90 | 0 | 0 | 19 | 1 | 35 | 51 | low |
| 74 | 1 | 0 | 15 | 1 | 30 | 68 | med |
| 94 | 0 | 0 | 20 | 1 | 1 | 52 | low |
| 127 | 8 | 1 | 12 | 0 | 513 | 40 | low |
| 190 | 8 | 4 | 17 | 4 | 330 | 47 | low |

# PASTA & NOODLES

| FOOD | SERVING SIZE | HOUSEHOLD MEASURE |
|---|---|---|
| Lasagne sheets, fresh | 2½ oz | 2 sheets |
| Linguine, thick, durum wheat, boiled | 2 oz | ⅓ cup |
| Linguine, thin, durum wheat, boiled | 2 oz | ⅓ cup |
| Macaroni, white, durum wheat, boiled | 2 oz | ⅓ cup |
| Macaroni and cheese, from packet mix, Kraft | 2½ oz | ⅛ packet |
| @ Maggi 2 Minute Noodles, Beef | 4¼ oz | ⅓ pack |
| @ Maggi 2 Minute Noodles, Chicken | 4¼ oz | ⅓ pack |
| @ Maggi 2 Minute Noodles, Curry | 4¼ oz | ⅓ pack |
| @ Maggi 2 Minute Noodles, Oriental | 4¼ oz | ⅓ pack |
| @ Maggi 2 Minute Noodles, Tomato | 4¼ oz | ⅓ pack |
| Mediterranean pasta sauce | 6 oz | I serving |
| Mung bean noodles, dried, boiled | 1¾ oz | ⅓ cup |
| Noodles, dried rice, boiled | 2½ oz | ⅓ cup |
| Noodles, fresh rice, boiled | 2½ oz | ⅓ cup |
| President's Choice® Blue Menu™ 100% Whole Wheat Lasagna pasta | 3 oz | 4 sheets |
| President's Choice ® Blue Menu™ 100% Whole Wheat Penne Rigate pasta | 3¼ oz | ⅕ package |
| President's Choice ® Blue Menu™ 100% Whole Wheat Spaghetti pasta | 3¼ oz | ⅕ package |

@ part of GI symbol program     ★ little or no carbs

| CALORIES | FAT (g) | SATURATED FAT (g) | CARBO-HYDRATE (g) | FIBER (g) | SODIUM (mg) | GI | LOW MED HIGH |
|---|---|---|---|---|---|---|---|
| 137 | 3 | 1 | 22 | 6 | 4 | 49 | low |
| 74 | 0 | 0 | 15 | 1 | 34 | 46 | low |
| 74 | 0 | 0 | 15 | 1 | 34 | 52 | low |
| 74 | 0 | 0 | 15 | 1 | 34 | 47 | low |
| 138 | 5 | 4 | 19 | 1 | 186 | 64 | med |
| 89 | 0 | 0 | 18 | 1 | 388 | 52 | low |
| 125 | 5 | 1 | 16 | 1 | 331 | 52 | low |
| 126 | 5 | 1 | 16 | 1 | 344 | 52 | low |
| 126 | 5 | 1 | 16 | 1 | 394 | 52 | low |
| 126 | 5 | 1 | 16 | 1 | 350 | 52 | low |
| 130 | 7 | 1 | 8 | 0 | 602 | 40 | low |
| 53 | 0 | 0 | 13 | 1 | 2 | 33 | low |
| 75 | 0 | 0 | 16 | 0 | 11 | 61 | med |
| 81 | 0 | 0 | 17 | 0 | 11 | 40 | low |
| 310 | 2 | 0 | 63 | 7 | 2 | 46 | low |
| 330 | 2 | 1 | 65 | 9 | 2 | 51 | low |
| 330 | 2 | 1 | 65 | 9 | 85 | 45 | low |

# PASTA & NOODLES

| FOOD | SERVING SIZE | HOUSEHOLD MEASURE |
|---|---|---|
| President's Choice® Blue Menu™ 100% Whole Wheat Spaghettini | 3¼ oz | ⅕ package |
| President's Choice® Blue Menu™ Fettuccini | 4 oz | ⅓ package |
| President's Choice® Blue Menu™ Whole Grain Lasagna Sheets | 2¼ oz | 1½ sheets |
| President's Choice® Blue Menu™ whole wheat rotini | 3 oz | ⅕ pack |
| Ravioli, meat-filled, durum wheat flour, boiled | 2 oz | ⅓ cup |
| Rice and corn pasta, gluten-free | 2½ oz | ⅓ cup |
| Rice pasta, brown, boiled | 5 oz | 1 cup |
| Rice vermicelli noodles, dried, boiled, Chinese | 2 oz | ⅓ cup |
| Ricotta & spinach agnolotti, fresh, commercially made | 5 oz | 1 serving |
| Soba noodles / buckwheat noodles | 4 oz | 1 cup |
| Soba noodles, instant, served in soup | 1¾ oz | ⅓ cup |
| Spaghetti with meat sauce, homemade | 5 oz | 1 serving |
| Spaghetti, gluten-free, canned in tomato sauce | 4 oz | ½ can |
| Spaghetti, protein-enriched, boiled | 1¾ oz | ⅓ cup |
| Spaghetti, white, durum wheat, boiled 10–15 mins | 2 oz | ⅓ cup |

| CALORIES | FAT (g) | SATURATED FAT (g) | CARBO-HYDRATE (g) | FIBER (g) | SODIUM (mg) | GI | LOW MED HIGH |
|---|---|---|---|---|---|---|---|
| 320 | 1 | 0 | 56 | 4 | 0 | 56 | med |
| 340 | 4 | 1 | 62 | 6 | 25 | 55 | low |
| 200 | 3 | 1 | 34 | 4 | 35 | 52 | low |
| 330 | 2 | 1 | 56 | 9 | 85 | 57 | med |
| 114 | 4 | 2 | 13 | 3 | 228 | 39 | low |
| 99 | 0 | 0 | 16 | 0 | 46 | 76 | high |
| 210 | 2 | 1 | 41 | 3 | 5 | 92 | high |
| 75 | 0 | 0 | 16 | 0 | 4 | 58 | med |
| 279 | 8 | 5 | 41 | 3 | 494 | 47 | low |
| 113 | 0 | 0 | 24 | 2 | 68 | 59 | med |
| 62 | 0 | 0 | 14 | 1 | 5 | 46 | low |
| 197 | 6 | 2 | 23 | 4 | 360 | 52 | low |
| 69 | 0 | 0 | 14 | 1 | 440 | 68 | med |
| 77 | 0 | 0 | 15 | 1 | 2 | 27 | low |
| 74 | 0 | 0 | 15 | 1 | 34 | 44 | low |

# PASTA & NOODLES

| FOOD | SERVING SIZE | HOUSEHOLD MEASURE |
|---|---|---|
| Spaghetti, whole wheat, boiled | 2 oz | ⅓ cup |
| Spicy tomato & bacon pasta sauce | 6 oz | 1 serve |
| Spirali, white, durum wheat, boiled | 2 oz | ⅓ cup |
| Toasted pasta, Osem brand, boiled | 2.2 oz | ½ cup |
| Udon noodles, plain, boiled | 2 oz | ⅓ cup |
| Veal tortellini, fresh, commercially made | 5 oz | 1 serving |
| Vermicelli pasta, white, durum wheat, boiled | 2 oz | ⅓ cup |
| Wholegrain ricotta & spinach ravioli, fresh, commercially made | 5 oz | 1 serving |

@ part of GI symbol program   ★ little or no carbs

| CALORIES | FAT (g) | SATURATED FAT (g) | CARBO-HYDRATE (g) | FIBER (g) | SODIUM (mg) | GI | LOW MED HIGH |
|---|---|---|---|---|---|---|---|
| 74 | 0 | 0 | 15 | 1 | 34 | 42 | low |
| 121 | 5 | 1 | 13 | 0 | 708 | 24 | low |
| 74 | 0 | 0 | 15 | 1 | 34 | 43 | low |
| 94 | 0 | 0 | 20 | 1 | 1 | 52 | low |
| 66 | 1 | 0 | 13 | 0 | 95 | 62 | med |
| 246 | 6 | 2 | 37 | 3 | 437 | 48 | low |
| 74 | 0 | 0 | 15 | 1 | 34 | 35 | low |
| 276 | 8 | 5 | 37 | 6 | 734 | 39 | low |

# RICE

| FOOD | SERVING SIZE | HOUSEHOLD MEASURE |
|---|---|---|
| Arborio risotto rice, white, boiled, SunRice® | 6.5 oz | 1 cup |
| Basmati rice, white, boiled | 5.5 oz | 1 cup |
| Broken rice, Thai, white, cooked in rice cooker | 6.5 oz | 1 cup |
| Brown Pelde rice, boiled | 6.75 oz | 1 cup |
| Calrose rice, brown, medium-grain, boiled | 6.75 oz | 1 cup |
| Calrose rice, white, medium-grain, boiled | 6.5 oz | 1 cup |
| Doongara Clever rice, Sunrice® | 5.5 oz | 1 cup |
| Doongara rice, brown, Sunrice® | 6.75 oz | 1 cup |
| Glutinous rice, white, cooked in rice cooker | 6 oz | 1 cup |
| Instant rice, white, cooked 6 mins with water | 6 oz | 1 cup |
| Jasmine fragrant rice, Sunrice® | 6 oz | 1 cup |
| Jasmine rice, white, long-grain, cooked in rice cooker | 6 oz | 1 cup |
| Long-grain rice, white, Mahatma®, boiled 15 mins | 5.5 oz | 1 cup |
| Moolgiri rice | 5.5 oz | 1 cup |
| Pelde parboiled rice, Sungold | 6 oz | 1 cup |
| Sunbrown Quick® rice, Ricegrowers, boiled | 6.5 oz | 1 cup |
| Sunrice® Japanese-Style Sushi Rice, white | 6 oz | 1 cup |

@ part of GI symbol program    ★ little or no carbs

| CALORIES | FAT (g) | SATURATED FAT (g) | CARBO-HYDRATE (g) | FIBER (g) | SODIUM (mg) | GI | LOW MED HIGH |
|---|---|---|---|---|---|---|---|
| 242 | 0 | 0 | 53 | 1 | 50 | 69 | med |
| 205 | 0 | 0 | 45 | 1 | 50 | 58 | med |
| 242 | 0 | 0 | 52 | 1 | 40 | 86 | high |
| 218 | 2 | 0 | 46 | 4 | 35 | 76 | high |
| 218 | 2 | 0 | 46 | 4 | 33 | 87 | high |
| 242 | 0 | 0 | 53 | 1 | 33 | 83 | high |
| 205 | 0 | 0 | 45 | 1 | 45 | 54 | low |
| 218 | 2 | 0 | 46 | 4 | 35 | 66 | med |
| 169 | 0 | 0 | 37 | 2 | 45 | 98 | high |
| 199 | 1 | 0 | 43 | 1 | 45 | 87 | high |
| 213 | 0 | 0 | 48 | 1 | 48 | 89 | high |
| 213 | 0 | 0 | 48 | 1 | 48 | 109 | high |
| 205 | 0 | 0 | 45 | 1 | 45 | 50 | low |
| 205 | 0 | 0 | 45 | 1 | 45 | 54 | low |
| 219 | 0 | 0 | 48 | 1 | 43 | 87 | high |
| 275 | 2 | 0 | 57 | 3 | 38 | 80 | high |
| 197 | 0 | 0 | 47 | 1 | 30 | 85 | high |

# RICE

| FOOD | SERVING SIZE | HOUSEHOLD MEASURE |
|------|------|------|
| Sunrice® Koshihikari rice, Ricegrowers | 6 oz | I cup |
| Sunrice® Medium Grain brown rice | 6.75 oz | I cup |
| Sunrice® Medium Grain Brown Rice in 90 seconds, microwaved | 4½ oz | ½ cup |
| Sunrice® Medium Grain white rice, boiled | 6 oz | I cup |
| Sunrice® Long Grain White Rice in 90 Seconds, microwaved | 4½ oz | ½ cup |
| Sunrice® Premium White Long Grain rice | 5.5 oz | I cup |
| Uncle Ben's® Original Converted, white | 5.5 oz | I cup (dry) |
| Uncle Ben's® Converted, white, boiled 20–30 min | 5.5 oz | I cup (dry) |
| Uncle Ben's® Converted, white, long grain, boiled 20–30 min | 5.5 oz | I cup (dry) |
| Uncle Ben's® Ready Rice® Whole Grain Brown Rice (pouch) | 5 oz | ⅔ cup |
| Uncle Ben's® Ready Rice® Whole Grain Chicken Flavored Brown Rice (pouch) | 5¼ oz | ⅔ cup |
| Uncle Ben's ® Ready Rice ® Long Grain & Wild (pouch) | 5 oz | ⅔ cup |
| Uncle Ben's ® Ready Rice ® Original Long Grain (pouch) | 5 oz | ⅔ cup |

＠ part of GI symbol program   ★ little or no carbs

| CALORIES | FAT (g) | SATURATED FAT (g) | CARBO-HYDRATE (g) | FIBER (g) | SODIUM (mg) | GI | LOW MED HIGH |
|---|---|---|---|---|---|---|---|
| 213 | 0 | 0 | 48 | 1 | 48 | 73 | high |
| 218 | 2 | 0 | 46 | 4 | 33 | 59 | med |
| 236 | 4 | 1 | 43 | 4 | 2 | 59 | med |
| 221 | 0 | 0 | 49 | 0 | 45 | 75 | high |
| 251 | 4 | 1 | 49 | 1 | 2 | 76 | high |
| 205 | 0 | 0 | 45 | 1 | 45 | 59 | med |
| 205 | 0 | 0 | 44 | 1 | 35 | 45 | low |
| 205 | 0 | 0 | 44 | 1 | 35 | 38 | low |
| 205 | 0 | 0 | 44 | 1 | 35 | 50 | low |
| 220 | 4 | 1 | 39 | 2 | 5 | 48 | low |
| 230 | 5 | 1 | 39 | 2 | 800 | 46 | low |
| 240 | 4 | 0 | 43 | 1 | 500 | 52 | low |
| 230 | 4 | 0 | 43 | 1 | 500 | 48 | low |

# RICE

| FOOD | SERVING SIZE | HOUSEHOLD MEASURE |
|------|------|------|
| Uncle Ben's® Ready Rice® Roasted Chicken Flavored (pouch) | 5 oz | ⅔ cup |
| Uncle Ben's® Santa Fe, Ready Whole Grain Medley™ (pouch) | 5 oz | 1 cup |
| Uncle Ben's® Spanish Style, Ready Rice® (pouch) | 5 oz | 1 cup |
| Uncle Ben's® Vegetable Harvest, Ready Whole Grain Medley™ (pouch) | 5 oz | 1 cup |
| Wild rice, boiled | 5.5 oz | 1 cup |

@ part of GI symbol program     ★ little or no carbs

| CALORIES | FAT (g) | SATURATED FAT (g) | CARBO-HYDRATE (g) | FIBER (g) | SODIUM (mg) | GI | LOW MED HIGH |
|---|---|---|---|---|---|---|---|
| 230 | 4 | 0 | 43 | 1 | 960 | 51 | low |
| 240 | 4 | 0 | 39 | 6 | 690 | 48 | low |
| 240 | 4 | 0 | 43 | 1 | 500 | 51 | low |
| 220 | 4 | 0 | 37 | 5 | 660 | 48 | low |
| 166 | 1 | 0 | 35 | 3 | 25 | 57 | med |

# SNACK FOODS

| FOOD | SERVING SIZE | HOUSEHOLD MEASURE |
|------|------|------|
| Apricot-filled fruit bar, wholemeal pastry | 1 oz | 1 bar |
| Cadbury's® milk chocolate, plain | 1 oz | 1 row |
| Cashew nuts, salted | 1¾ oz | ⅓ cup |
| Chickpea chips | 2 oz | 1 small packet |
| Chocolate #9 (gourmet chocolate sauce, sweetened w/ agave) | 1 oz | 2 tbsp |
| Chocolate brownies | 2 oz | 1 large brownie |
| Chocolate, dark, Dove® | 1 oz | ⅓ bar |
| Chocolate, dark, plain, regular | 1 oz | 1 row family-sized block |
| Chocolate, milk, plain, Nestlé® | 1 oz | 1 row |
| Chocolate, milk, plain, reduced sugar | 1 oz | 1 row |
| Chocolate, milk, plain, regular | 1 oz | 1 row |
| Chocolate, milk, plain, with fructose instead of regular sugar | 1 oz | 1 row |
| Chocolate candy, sugar free, Dove® | 1.2 oz | ⅓ bar |
| Chocolate Raspberry Zing™ bar, Revival Soy® | 1 bar | 1 bar |
| Cinch™ Chocolate weight management bar, Shaklee Corporation | 1 oz | 1 bar |

ⓖ part of GI symbol program    ★ little or no carbs

| CALORIES | FAT (g) | SATURATED FAT (g) | CARBO-HYDRATE (g) | FIBER (g) | SODIUM (mg) | GI | LOW MED HIGH |
|---|---|---|---|---|---|---|---|
| 105 | 5 | 4 | 12 | 6 | 25 | 50 | low |
| 147 | 8 | 5 | 16 | 1 | 36 | 49 | low |
| 319 | 26 | 4 | 13 | 2 | 145 | 22 | low |
| 245 | 12 | 3 | 25 | 6 | 22 | 44 | low |
| 70 | 1 | 0 | 15 | 1 | 75 | 46 | low |
| 227 | 9 | 2 | 36 | 1 | 175 | 42 | low |
| 170 | 11 | 5 | 23 | 3 | 0 | 23 | low |
| 144 | 9 | 8 | 16 | 1 | 13 | 41 | low |
| 145 | 8 | 5 | 17 | 0 | 25 | 42 | low |
| 108 | 8 | 5 | 17 | 0 | 25 | 35 | low |
| 145 | 8 | 5 | 17 | 0 | 25 | 41 | low |
| 145 | 8 | 5 | 17 | 0 | 25 | 20 | low |
| 149 | 11 | 5 | 14 | 3 | 0 | 23 | low |
| 230 | 7 | 4 | 10 | 5 | 280 | 47 | low |
| 120 | 3 | 1 | 15 | 3 | 170 | 29 | low |

# SNACK FOODS

| FOOD | SERVING SIZE | HOUSEHOLD MEASURE |
|------|------|------|
| Cinch™ Lemon Cranberry weight management bar, Shaklee Corporation | 1 oz | 1 bar |
| Cinch™ Peanut Butter weight management bar, Shaklee Corporation | 1 oz | 1 bar |
| Clif bar, Chocolate Brownie Energy bar | 2¼ oz | 1 bar |
| Clif Bar, Cookies 'n Cream | 2¼ oz | 1 bar |
| CocoaVia Chocolate Almond Snack Bar | ¾ oz | 1 bar |
| CocoaVia Chocolate Covered Almonds | 1 oz | 1 pack |
| CocoaVia Crispy Chocolate Bar | ¾ oz | 1 bar |
| Combos® Snacks Cheddar Cheese Crackers | 1¾ oz | 1 bag |
| Combos® Snacks Cheddar Cheese Pretzels | 1¾ oz | 1 bag |
| Corn chips, Nachips™ | 1 oz | 8 chips |
| Corn chips, plain, salted | 1 oz | 15 chips |
| Dove® milk chocolate | 1 oz | ⅓ bar |
| ExtendBar™ Apple Cinnamon Delight Bar | 1.35 oz | 1 bar |
| ExtendBar™ Chocolate Delight Bar | 1.35 oz | 1 bar |
| ExtendBar™ Peanut Delight Bar | 1.35 oz | 1 bar |
| Fruit and nut mix | 2 oz | 1 small handful |

@ part of GI symbol program      ★ little or no carbs

| CALORIES | FAT (g) | SATURATED FAT (g) | CARBO-HYDRATE (g) | FIBER (g) | SODIUM (mg) | GI | LOW MED HIGH |
|---|---|---|---|---|---|---|---|
| 120 | 3 | 1 | 15 | 3 | 150 | 23 | low |
| 120 | 3 | 1 | 15 | 3 | 190 | 22 | low |
| 240 | 5 | 2 | 45 | 5 | 150 | 57 | med |
| 240 | 4 | 2 | 42 | 5 | 180 | 101 | high |
| 80 | 2 | 1 | 12 | 1 | 60 | 63 | med |
| 140 | 11 | 4 | 9 | 3 | 0 | 21 | low |
| 90 | 5 | 3 | 9 | 2 | 10 | 33 | low |
| 240 | 11 | 5 | 30 | 1 | 490 | 54 | low |
| 240 | 8 | 5 | 33 | 1 | 790 | 52 | low |
| 150 | 8 | 2 | 17 | 2 | 85 | 74 | high |
| 140 | 8 | 3 | 17 | 3 | 138 | 42 | low |
| 158 | 9 | 6 | 17 | 1 | 56 | 45 | low |
| 150 | 2 | 0 | 21 | 5 | 135 | 33 | low |
| 150 | 3 | 2 | 21 | 5 | 170 | 41 | low |
| 150 | 3 | 1 | 21 | 5 | 160 | 32 | low |
| 233 | 12 | 3 | 25 | 4 | 27 | 32 | low |

# SNACK FOODS

| FOOD | SERVING SIZE | HOUSEHOLD MEASURE |
|------|------|------|
| Gummi confectionary, based on glucose syrup | ¾ oz | 5 pieces |
| Ironman PR bar®, chocolate | 1½ oz | 1 bar |
| Jell-O, Raspberry flavor | 4 oz | ½ cup |
| Jelly beans | ¾ oz | 6 pieces |
| K-Time® Just Right® breakfast cereal bar | ½ oz | ½ bar |
| Kudos Milk Chocolate Granola Bars, Peanut Butter Flavor | 1 oz | 1 bar |
| Kudos Milk Chocolate Granola Bars, with M&M's | ¾ oz | 1 bar |
| Licorice, soft | 1 oz | 2 pieces |
| Life Savers®, peppermint | ½ oz | ¾ roll |
| Luna Protein Chocolate Peanut Butter Bar | 1½ oz | 1 bar |
| Luna Cookie Dough Bar | 1½ oz | 1 bar |
| Mars Bar®, regular | 1 oz | 1 funsize bar |
| Marshmallows, plain, pink and white | ½ oz | 4 round pieces |
| Milky Bar®, white, Nestlé® | 1 oz | 2 mini-bars |
| Milky Way Bar | 2 oz | 1 bar |
| M&M's®, peanut | 1 oz | ½ packet |
| Muesli bar, chewy, with choc chips or fruit | 1 oz | ¾ bar |
| Muesli bar, crunchy, with dried fruit | ¾ oz | 1 bar |
| Munch Peanut Butter bar, M&M/Mars | 1.35 oz | 1 bar |

| CALORIES | FAT (g) | SATURATED FAT (g) | CARBO-HYDRATE (g) | FIBER (g) | SODIUM (mg) | GI | LOW MED HIGH |
|---|---|---|---|---|---|---|---|
| 63 | 0 | 0 | 15 | 0 | 3 | 94 | high |
| 190 | 6 | 3 | 19 | 0 | 130 | 39 | low |
| 80 | 0 | 0 | 18 | 0 | 6 | 53 | low |
| 62 | 0 | 0 | 15 | 0 | 25 | 78 | high |
| 62 | 1 | 0 | 13 | 1 | 4 | 72 | high |
| 130 | 6 | 3 | 17 | 1 | 75 | 45 | low |
| 100 | 3 | 2 | 16 | 1 | 80 | 52 | low |
| 61 | 0 | 0 | 14 | 1 | 31 | 78 | high |
| 65 | 0 | 0 | 16 | 0 | 1 | 70 | high |
| 190 | 9 | 4 | 19 | 2 | 210 | 28 | low |
| 180 | 6 | 4 | 21 | 3 | 230 | 18 | low |
| 114 | 4 | 3 | 18 | 0 | 37 | 62 | med |
| 48 | 0 | 0 | 15 | 0 | 5 | 62 | med |
| 168 | 10 | 6 | 17 | 0 | 35 | 44 | low |
| 260 | 10 | 7 | 40 | 1 | 95 | 62 | med |
| 142 | 8 | 3 | 17 | 0 | 15 | 33 | low |
| 98 | 3 | 1 | 15 | 0 | 60 | 54 | low |
| 85 | 2 | 0 | 14 | 0 | 64 | 61 | med |
| 286 | 19 | 4 | 22 | 3 | 65 | 27 | low |

# SNACK FOODS

| FOOD | SERVING SIZE | HOUSEHOLD MEASURE |
|------|------|------|
| NutriSystem®, Apple Cinnamon Soy Chips | 1 oz | 1 container |
| NutriSystem® Apple Granola bar | 1.4 oz | 1 bar |
| NutriSystem®, Blueberry Dessert Bar | 1½ oz | 1 container |
| NutriSystem®, Chocolate Crunch Bar | 1 oz | 1 container |
| NutriSystem®, Chocolate | 1½ oz | 1 container |
| NutriSystem® Cinnamon Swirl Granola bar | 1.4 oz | 1 bar |
| NutriSystem® Cranberry Granola bar | 1.4 oz | 1 bar |
| NutriSystem® Fudge Brownie | 1.2 oz | 1 brownie |
| NutriSystem® Honey Mustard Pretzels | 1 oz | 1 container |
| NutriSystem® Peanut Butter Granola bar | | 1 bar |
| Nuts, mixed, roasted and salted | ½ oz | 1 tbsp |
| Peanut Butter Chocolate Buddy™ bar, Revival Soy® | 1 bar | 1 bar |
| Performance Chocolate energy bar, Power Bar | 2.2 oz | 1 bar |
| Peanuts, roasted, salted | 5½ oz | 1 cup |
| Pecan nuts, raw | ½ oz | 1 tbsp |
| Pirate's Booty®, Aged White Cheddar snack | 1 oz | 1 package |

@ part of GI symbol program   ★ little or no carbs

| CALORIES | FAT (g) | SATURATED FAT (g) | CARBO-HYDRATE (g) | FIBER (g) | SODIUM (mg) | GI | LOW MED HIGH |
|---|---|---|---|---|---|---|---|
| 110 | 3 | 0 | 10 | 2 | 135 | 36 | low |
| 150 | 2 | 0 | 28 | 2 | 50 | 52 | low |
| 140 | 4 | 3 | 21 | 3 | 115 | 36 | low |
| 130 | 6 | 5 | 15 | 0 | 130 | 41 | low |
| 180 | 8 | 3 | 18 | 2 | 170 | 48 | low |
| 150 | 2 | 0 | 27 | 2 | 55 | 47 | low |
| 150 | 2 | 0 | 27 | 2 | 45 | 50 | low |
| 140 | 5 | 1 | 22 | 6 | 230 | 41 | low |
| 140 | 6 | 2 | 7 | 3 | 330 | 32 | low |
| 170 | 6 | 1 | 18 | 2 | 125 | 32 | low |
| 84 | 7 | 1 | 4 | 1 | 95 | 24 | low |
| 260 | 7 | 1 | 30 | 5 | 320 | 52 | low |
| 230 | 2 | 1 | 44 | 4 | 200 | 53 | low |
| 871 | 72 | 8 | 14 | 13 | 900 | 14 | low |
| 93 | 9 | 1 | 2 | 1 | 10 | ★ | |
| 130 | 5 | 1 | 19 | 0 | 140 | 70 | high |

# SNACK FOODS

| FOOD | SERVING SIZE | HOUSEHOLD MEASURE |
|------|------|------|
| Pop-Tarts®, double chocolate | 1 oz | ½ tart |
| Popcorn, plain, cooked in microwave | 1 oz | 3 cups |
| Potato chips, plain, salted | 1¾ oz | 30 chips |
| PowerBar®, Chocolate | 2 oz | 1 bar |
| President's Choice® Blue Menu™ 60% Whole Wheat Fig Fruit bar | 1.35 oz | 2 bars |
| President's Choice® Blue Menu™ Apple Fruit Bar, Fat-Free | 1.35 oz | 2 bars |
| President's Choice® Blue Menu™ Chewy Chocolate Chip & Marshmallow Granola Bar | 0.9 oz | 1 bar |
| President's Choice® Blue Menu™ Chewy Cranberry Apple Granola Bar | 0.9 oz | 1 bar |
| President's Choice® Blue Menu™ Fig Fruit bar | 1.35 oz | 2 bars |
| President's Choice® Blue Menu™ Flaxseed Tortilla Chips, Sea Salt | 1¾ oz | 17 chips |
| President's Choice® Blue Menu™ Flaxseed Tortilla Chips, Spicy | 1¾ oz | 17 chips |
| President's Choice® Blue Menu™ Fruit & Nut Bar, Apple & Almonds | 1 oz | 1 bar |
| President's Choice® Blue Menu™ Fruit & Nut Mixed Berries & Almonds Chewy Multi-Grain Bars | 1¼ oz | 1 bar |

@ part of GI symbol program   ★ little or no carbs

| CALORIES | FAT (g) | SATURATED FAT (g) | CARBO-HYDRATE (g) | FIBER (g) | SODIUM (mg) | GI | LOW MED HIGH |
|---|---|---|---|---|---|---|---|
| 101 | 2 | 1 | 19 | 0 | 101 | 70 | high |
| 89 | 1 | 0 | 14 | 6 | 1 | 72 | high |
| 271 | 19 | 5 | 27 | 2 | 260 | 51 | low |
| 230 | 2 | 1 | 40 | 4 | 200 | 53 | low |
| 130 | 0 | 0 | 31 | 2 | 110 | 72 | high |
| 130 | 0 | 0 | 31 | 1 | 115 | 90 | high |
| 110 | 2 | 1 | 21 | 1 | 50 | 78 | high |
| 100 | 2 | 0 | 21 | 1 | 55 | 58 | med |
| 130 | 0 | 0 | 31 | 1 | 110 | 70 | high |
| 250 | 14 | 2 | 20 | 6 | 170 | 64 | med |
| 250 | 14 | 2 | 20 | 6 | 370 | 64 | med |
| 130 | 3 | 0 | 20 | 5 | 90 | 65 | med |
| 140 | 3 | 0 | 26 | 5 | 95 | 63 | med |

# SNACK FOODS

| FOOD | SERVING SIZE | HOUSEHOLD MEASURE |
|------|------|------|
| President's Choice® Blue Menu™ Fruit & Yogurt Apple Cinnamon Chewy Bars (Soy) | 1½ oz | 1 bar |
| President's Choice® Blue Menu™ Fruit & Yogurt Cranberry Blueberry Bars (Soy) | 1½ oz | 1 bar |
| President's Choice® Blue Menu™ Japanese Wasabi & Honey Rice & Corn Crisps | 1¾ oz | 30 chips |
| President's Choice® Blue Menu™ Microwave Popping Corn, butter flavor | 1½ oz | 6 cups popped |
| President's Choice® Blue Menu™ Microwave Popping Corn, natural flavor | 1½ oz | 6 cups popped |
| President's Choice® Blue Menu™ Original & Tomato Basil Vegetable Sticks | 1¾ oz | ½ package |
| President's Choice® Blue Menu™ Raspberry Fruit bar, fat-free | 1.35 oz | 2 bars |
| President's Choice® Blue Menu™ Rice & Corn Chips, Japanese Tamari | 1 ¾ oz | 30 chips |
| President's Choice® Blue Menu™ Rice & Corn Chips, Thai Curry | 1¾ oz | 30 chips |
| President's Choice® Blue Menu™ Two-Bite Brownie | 1¼ oz | 2 brownies |
| Pretzels, oven-baked, traditional wheat flavor | ¾ oz | 1 small packet |

@ part of GI symbol program ★ little or no carbs

| CALORIES | FAT (g) | SATURATED FAT (g) | CARBO-HYDRATE (g) | FIBER (g) | SODIUM (mg) | GI | LOW MED HIGH |
|---|---|---|---|---|---|---|---|
| 170 | 5 | 2 | 21 | 2 | 170 | 34 | low |
| 170 | 5 | 2 | 21 | 2 | 130 | 33 | low |
| 200 | 3 | 0 | 40 | 1 | 600 | 82 | high |
| 160 | 3 | 1 | 31 | 5 | 230 | 72 | high |
| 160 | 3 | 1 | 31 | 5 | 230 | 58 | med |
| 200 | 4 | 1 | 38 | 1 | 700 | 65 | med |
| 130 | 0 | 0 | 32 | 1 | 105 | 74 | high |
| 200 | 3 | 0 | 38 | 1 | 470 | 91 | high |
| 200 | 3 | 0 | 39 | 2 | 550 | 84 | high |
| 150 | 6 | 2 | 23 | 4 | 110 | 62 | med |
| 76 | 1 | 0 | 13 | 1 | 396 | 83 | high |

# SNACK FOODS

| FOOD | SERVING SIZE | HOUSEHOLD MEASURE |
|------|------|------|
| Rice Krispie Treat® bar, Kellogg's® | ¾ oz | 1 bar |
| Roll-Ups®, processed fruit snack | ¾ oz | 1 |
| Skittles® | ¾ oz | 5 pieces |
| SlimFast® Meal Options bar, rich chocolate brownie flavor | 2 oz | 1 bar |
| SmartZone Chocolate Flavor Nutrition bar | 1.7 oz | 1 bar |
| SmartZone Crunchy Blueberry Flavor Nutrition Bar | 1.7 oz | 1 bar |
| SmartZone Crunchy Chocolate Brownie Flavor Nutrition Bar | 1.7 oz | 1 bar |
| SmartZone Crunchy Chocolate Caramel Flavor Nutrition Bar | 1.7 oz | 1 bar |
| SmartZone Crunchy Chocolate Peanut Butter Flavor Nutrition Bar | 1.7 oz | 1 bar |
| SmartZone Crunchy Key Lime Flavor Nutrition Bar | 1.7 oz | 1 bar |
| SmartZone Peanut Butter Flavor Nutrition Bar | 1.7 oz | 1 bar |
| Snickers® Bar | 2 oz | 1 bar |
| Snickers® Marathon Energy Bar, Cookies & Crème flavor | 1.85 oz | 1 bar |
| Snickers® Marathon Nutrition Bar, Dark Chocolate Crunch flavor | 1.4 oz | 1 bar |
| Snickers® Marathon Nutrition Bar, Honey & Toasted Almond flavor | 1.4 oz | 1 bar |

@ part of GI symbol program   ★ little or no carbs

| CALORIES | FAT (g) | SATURATED FAT (g) | CARBO-HYDRATE (g) | FIBER (g) | SODIUM (mg) | GI | LOW MED HIGH |
|---|---|---|---|---|---|---|---|
| 91 | 2 | 1 | 17 | 0 | 81 | 63 | med |
| 66 | 1 | 0 | 14 | 0 | 1 | 99 | high |
| 82 | 1 | 1 | 18 | 0 | 9 | 70 | high |
| 220 | 5 | 4 | 34 | 2 | 170 | 64 | med |
| 211 | 8 | 4 | 24 | 3 | 250 | 16 | low |
| 200 | 6 | 4 | 22 | 2 | 290 | 15 | low |
| 200 | 7 | 4 | 21 | 3 | 290 | 23 | low |
| 210 | 7 | 4 | 23 | 2 | 200 | 16 | low |
| 204 | 8 | 4 | 21 | 3 | 250 | 14 | low |
| 200 | 6 | 4 | 22 | 2 | 290 | 14 | low |
| 200 | 7 | 3 | 21 | 3 | 290 | 18 | low |
| 280 | 14 | 5 | 34 | 1 | 140 | 43 | low |
| 200 | 5 | 4 | 31 | 1 | 240 | 50 | low |
| 150 | 4 | 3 | 23 | 7 | 160 | 49 | low |
| 150 | 4 | 2 | 21 | 7 | 130 | 41 | low |

# SNACK FOODS

| FOOD | SERVING SIZE | HOUSEHOLD MEASURE |
|---|---|---|
| Snickers® Marathon Energy Bar, Peanut Butter flavor | 1.85 oz | 1 bar |
| Snickers® Marathon Low Carb Lifestyle Energy Bar, Chocolate Fudge Brownie Flavor | 1¾ oz | 1 bar |
| Snickers® Marathon Low Carb Lifestyle Energy Bar, Peanut Butter Flavor | 1¾ oz | 1 bar |
| Snickers® Marathon Protein Performance Bar, Caramel Nut Rush Flavor | 2¾ oz | 1 bar |
| Snickers® Marathon Protein Performance Bar, Chocolate Nut Burst Flavor | 2¾ oz | 1 bar |
| SoLo GI Nutrition Bar, Berry Bliss | 1¾ oz | 1 bar |
| SoLo GI Nutrition Bar, Chocolate Charger | 1¾ oz | 1 bar |
| SoLo GI Nutrition Bar, Mint Mania | 1¾ oz | 1 bar |
| SoLo GI Nutrition Bar, Peanut Power | 1¾ oz | 1 bar |
| SoLo GI Nutrition Bar, Lemon Lift | 1¾ oz | 1 bar |
| SoLo GI Snack Bar, Berry Bliss | 1 oz | 1 bar |
| SoLo GI Snack Bar, Chocolate Charger | 1 oz | 1 bar |
| SoLo GI Snack Bar, Mint Mania | 1 oz | 1 bar |
| SoLo GI Snack Bar, Peanut Power | 1 oz | 1 bar |
| SoLo GI Snack Bar, Lemon Lift | 1 oz | 1 bar |

@ part of GI symbol program    ★ little or no carbs

| CALORIES | FAT (g) | SATURATED FAT (g) | CARBO-HYDRATE (g) | FIBER (g) | SODIUM (mg) | GI | LOW MED HIGH |
|---|---|---|---|---|---|---|---|
| 210 | 8 | 4 | 25 | 4 | 240 | 34 | low |
| 170 | 7 | 3 | 11 | 8 | 240 | 20 | low |
| 160 | 6 | 2 | 11 | 7 | 260 | 21 | low |
| 290 | 8 | 4 | 33 | 8 | 180 | 26 | low |
| 290 | 7 | 3 | 29 | 7 | 260 | 32 | low |
| 200 | 6 | 3 | 22 | 3 | 125 | 28 | low |
| 200 | 7 | 3 | 22 | 4 | 120 | 28 | low |
| 200 | 7 | 3 | 22 | 4 | 120 | 23 | low |
| 200 | 8 | 3 | 20 | 3 | 125 | 27 | low |
| 200 | 6 | 3 | 22 | 4 | 105 | 28 | low |
| 100 | 3 | 2 | 11 | 2 | 60 | 28 | low |
| 100 | 3 | 2 | 10 | 2 | 60 | 28 | low |
| 100 | 3 | 2 | 10 | 2 | 60 | 23 | low |
| 100 | 4 | 2 | 10 | 2 | 60 | 27 | low |
| 100 | 3 | 2 | 11 | 2 | 55 | 28 | low |

# SNACK FOODS

| FOOD | SERVING SIZE | HOUSEHOLD MEASURE |
|------|------|------|
| Stretch Island Fruit Co™ Summer Strawberry fruit leather | ½ oz | 1 bar |
| ⓖ Sunripe School Straps Blackberry Sour Buzz | ¾ oz | 1½ bars |
| ⓖ Sunripe School Straps, dried fruit snack | ¾ oz | 1½ bars |
| Sunshine™ soy protein chips, lightly salted, Revival Soy® | 0.9 oz | 1 bag |
| Twisties®, cheese-flavored snack | 1 oz | ½ oz packet |
| Twix® bar | ½ oz | 1 fun-size bar |
| VO2 Max Chocolate Energy Bar, M&M/Mars | 2.2 oz | 1 bar |
| ZonePerfect® nutrition bar, double chocolate flavor | 1.7 oz | 1 bar |

| CALORIES | FAT (g) | SATURATED FAT (g) | CARBO-HYDRATE (g) | FIBER (g) | SODIUM (mg) | GI | LOW MED HIGH |
|---|---|---|---|---|---|---|---|
| 45 | 0 | 0 | 11 | 1 | 0 | 29 | low |
| 68 | 0 | 0 | 15 | 2 | 8 | 35 | low |
| 72 | 0 | 0 | 17 | 2 | 8 | 40 | low |
| 100 | 2 | 0 | 13 | 0 | 180 | 87 | high |
| 108 | 7 | 4 | 15 | 1 | 278 | 74 | high |
| 91 | 5 | 3 | 12 | 1 | 28 | 44 | low |
| 210 | 3 | 1 | 45 | 2 | 220 | 49 | low |
| 210 | 7 | 5 | 20 | 1 | 260 | 44 | low |

# SOUPS

| FOOD | SERVING SIZE | HOUSEHOLD MEASURE |
|------|------|------|
| Black bean, canned | 8 oz | I cup |
| Chicken and mushroom soup | 8 oz | I cup |
| Chicken and Vegetable with wholegrain pasta, Campbell's® | 8 oz | I cup |
| Clear consommé, chicken or vegetable | 8 fl oz | I cup |
| Green pea, canned | 9 oz | ½ can |
| Lentil, canned | 9 oz | I cup |
| Minestrone, traditional, | 9 oz | I cup |
| Campbell's® Minestrone, condensed, prepared with water | 8 oz | I cup |
| President's Choice® Blue Menu™ Barley Vegetable Low Fat Instant Soup | 9 oz | I container |
| President's Choice® Blue Menu™ Chicken & Rotini Soup | 9 oz | I container |
| President's Choice® Blue Menu™ Indian Lentil Low Fat Instant Soup | 9 oz | I container |
| President's Choice® Blue Menu™ Lentil Soup | 9 oz | I container |
| President's Choice® Blue Menu™ Minestrone & Pasta Instant soup, low-fat | 9 oz | I container |
| President's Choice® Blue Menu™ Mushroom Barley, Ready-to-Serve | 9 oz | I container |

@ part of GI symbol program   ★ little or no carbs

| CALORIES | FAT (g) | SATURATED FAT (g) | CARBO-HYDRATE (g) | FIBER (g) | SODIUM (mg) | GI | LOW MED HIGH |
|---|---|---|---|---|---|---|---|
| 108 | 1 | 0 | 18 | 4 | 1105 | 64 | med |
| 274 | 18 | 5 | 18 | 1 | 1940 | 58 | med |
| 86 | 2 | 0 | 11 | 2 | 739 | 43 | low |
| 17 | 0 | 0 | 2 | 0 | 1600 | ★ | |
| 180 | 7 | 4 | 19 | 5 | 613 | 66 | med |
| 98 | 1 | 0 | 13 | 5 | 867 | 44 | low |
| 140 | 4 | 1 | 13 | 10 | 520 | 39 | low |
| 180 | 2 | 1 | 28 | 6 | 1920 | 48 | low |
| 160 | 2 | 0 | 28 | 5 | 430 | 41 | low |
| 100 | 2 | 1 | 15 | 4 | 480 | 38 | low |
| 150 | 2 | 0 | 20 | 5 | 500 | 55 | low |
| 140 | 3 | 1 | 19 | 4 | 480 | 56 | med |
| 230 | 2 | 1 | 46 | 5 | 540 | 54 | low |
| 80 | 2 | 0 | 9 | 3 | 480 | 45 | low |

# SOUPS

| FOOD | SERVING SIZE | HOUSEHOLD MEASURE |
|------|------|------|
| President's Choice® Blue Menu™ Pasta e Fagioli Soup, Ready-to-Serve | 9 oz | I container |
| President's Choice® Blue Menu™ Soupreme, Carrot Soup | 9 oz | I container |
| President's Choice® Blue Menu™ Soupreme, Tomato and Herb Soup | 9 oz | I container |
| President's Choice® Blue Menu™ Soupreme, Winter Squash Soup | 9 oz | I container |
| President's Choice® Blue Menu™ Spicy Black Bean Low Fat Instant Soup | 9 oz | I container |
| President's Choice® Blue Menu™ Spicy Black Bean with Vegetables Soup | 9 oz | I container |
| President's Choice® Blue Menu™ Spicy Thai Instant Noodles with Vegetables Low Fat Instant Soup | 9 oz | I container |
| President's Choice® Blue Menu™ Vegetable CousCous Low Fat Instant Soup Cup | 9 oz | I container |
| President's Choice® Blue Menu™ Vegetarian Chili, Ready-to-Serve | 9 oz | I container |
| President's Choice® Blue Menu™ Vegetarian Chili Low Fat Instant Cup | 9 oz | I container |

@ part of GI symbol program     ★ little or no carbs

| CALORIES | FAT (g) | SATURATED FAT (g) | CARBO-HYDRATE (g) | FIBER (g) | SODIUM (mg) | GI | LOW MED HIGH |
|---|---|---|---|---|---|---|---|
| 160 | 3 | 1 | 20 | 5 | 480 | 52 | low |
| 100 | 3 | 0 | 13 | 3 | 420 | 35 | low |
| 80 | 1 | 0 | 14 | 2 | 340 | 47 | low |
| 90 | 2 | 1 | 15 | 5 | 542 | 41 | low |
| 240 | 1 | 0 | 32 | 13 | 680 | 57 | med |
| 200 | 3 | 0 | 34 | 7 | 480 | 46 | low |
| 170 | 1 | 0 | 31 | 6 | 250 | 56 | med |
| 200 | 1 | 0 | 33 | 6 | 510 | 57 | med |
| 200 | 3 | 1 | 29 | 5 | 480 | 39 | low |
| 230 | 2 | 0 | 29 | 11 | 420 | 36 | low |

# SOUPS

| FOOD | SERVING SIZE | HOUSEHOLD MEASURE |
|---|---|---|
| Pumpkin, Creamy, Heinz® | 7 oz | ½ can |
| Split pea, canned | 8 oz | 1 cup |
| Tomato, canned | 9 oz | 1 cup |
| Tomato soup, condensed, prepared with water, Campbell's® | 8 oz | 1 cup |
| Vegetable soup | 8 oz | 1 cup |

@ part of GI symbol program   ★ little or no carbs

| CALORIES | FAT (g) | SATURATED FAT (g) | CARBO-HYDRATE (g) | FIBER (g) | SODIUM (mg) | GI | LOW MED HIGH |
|---|---|---|---|---|---|---|---|
| 106 | 2 | 0 | 16 | 4 | 672 | 76 | high |
| 160 | 2 | 0 | 27 | 4 | 373 | 60 | med |
| 70 | 1 | 0 | 14 | 3 | 850 | 45 | low |
| 180 | 0 | 0 | 40 | 2 | 1420 | 52 | low |
| 125 | 4 | 1 | 18 | 1 | 880 | 60 | med |

# SOY PRODUCTS

| FOOD | SERVING SIZE | HOUSEHOLD MEASURE |
|---|---|---|
| ⓖ Bürgen® Soy-Lin Muesli | ¾ oz | ¼ cup |
| ⓖ Bürgen® Soy-Lin, soy and flaxseed bread | 1½ oz | 1 slice |
| ⓖ Country Life Rye Hi-soy and flaxseed bread | 1¾ oz | 1½ slices |
| Flaxseed and soy bread | 3 oz | 2 slices |
| NutriSystem®, Apple Cinnamon Soy Chips | 1 oz | 1 container |
| NutriSystem®, Sour Cream and Onion Soy Chips | 1 oz | 1 container |
| President's Choice® Blue Menu™ Popcorn, Microwave, Natural Flavor | 6 cups popped | ½ bag |
| President's Choice® Blue Menu™ Soy Beverage, Chocolate flavored | 8 fl oz | 1 cup |
| President's Choice® Blue Menu™ Soy Beverage, Original flavored | 8 fl oz | 1 cup |
| President's Choice® Blue Menu™ Soy Beverage, Vanilla flavored | 8 fl oz | 1 cup |
| ⓖ So Natural Calciforte, soy milk, calcium-enriched, full fat | 8 fl oz | 1 cup |
| So Natural Light, soy milk, reduced fat, calcium-fortified | 8 fl oz | 1 cup |
| So Natural Original, soy milk, full fat (3%) | 8 fl oz | 1 cup |
| Soy beans, canned, drained | 6 oz | 1 cup |

ⓖ part of GI symbol program   ★ little or no carbs

| CALORIES | FAT (g) | SATURATED FAT (g) | CARBO-HYDRATE (g) | FIBER (g) | SODIUM (mg) | GI | LOW MED HIGH |
|---|---|---|---|---|---|---|---|
| 92 | 3 | 0 | 13 | 3 | 37 | 51 | low |
| 97 | 3 | 0 | 12 | 2 | 146 | 36 | low |
| 111 | 2 | 0 | 14 | 5 | 110 | 42 | low |
| 230 | 8 | 1 | 26 | 6 | 364 | 55 | low |
| 110 | 3 | 0 | 10 | 2 | 135 | 36 | low |
| 110 | 3 | 0 | 10 | 2 | 320 | 41 | low |
| 160 | 3 | 1 | 25 | 4 | 200 | 58 | med |
| 160 | 3 | 1 | 28 | 0 | 140 | 40 | low |
| 90 | 3 | 1 | 9 | 0 | 150 | 15 | low |
| 120 | 3 | 1 | 16 | 0 | 160 | 28 | low |
| 172 | 7 | 1 | 19 | 1 | 233 | 40 | low |
| 105 | 1 | 0 | 14 | 1 | 98 | 44 | low |
| 158 | 7 | 1 | 19 | 1 | 225 | 44 | low |
| 169 | 9 | 1 | 5 | 8 | 629 | 14 | low |

# SOY PRODUCTS

| FOOD | SERVING SIZE | HOUSEHOLD MEASURE |
|------|------|------|
| Soy beans, dried, boiled | 6 oz | 1 cup |
| Soy yogurt, Peach and Mango, 2% fat, with sugar | 3½ oz | ½ container |
| Vitasoy® Light Original, soy milk | 12 fl oz | 1½ cups |
| Vitasoy® Lush, chocolate, reduced fat soy milk | 8 fl oz | 1 cup |
| Vitasoy® Lush, vanilla, reduced fat soy milk | 8 fl oz | 1 cup |
| Vitasoy® Organic soy milk | 8 fl oz | 1 cup |
| Vitasoy® Premium Calci Plus® High Fiber, soy milk, 98.5% fat free | 8 fl oz | 1 cup |
| Vitasoy® Premium Calci Plus®, soy milk | 8 fl oz | 1 cup |
| Vitasoy® Soy Milky, regular, soy milk | 8 fl oz | 1 cup |
| Vitasoy® Soy Milky, lite, soy milk | 8 fl oz | 1 cup |

@ part of GI symbol program   ★ little or no carbs

| CALORIES | FAT (g) | SATURATED FAT (g) | CARBO-HYDRATE (g) | FIBER (g) | SODIUM (mg) | GI | LOW MED HIGH |
|---|---|---|---|---|---|---|---|
| 242 | 13 | 2 | 2 | 12 | 15 | 18 | low |
| 69 | 2 | 0 | 8 | 1 | 58 | 50 | low |
| 106 | 3 | 0 | 15 | 0 | 161 | 45 | low |
| 139 | 4 | 1 | 19 | 1 | 218 | 31 | low |
| 128 | 4 | 1 | 16 | 1 | 165 | 31 | low |
| 120 | 4 | 1 | 16 | 3 | 30 | 43 | low |
| 121 | 4 | 1 | 14 | 4 | 110 | 16 | low |
| 160 | 8 | 2 | 15 | 1 | 120 | 24 | med |
| 132 | 8 | 1 | 8 | 1 | 225 | 21 | low |
| 95 | 4 | 1 | 7 | 1 | 225 | 17 | low |

# SPREADS & SWEETENERS

| FOOD | SERVING SIZE | HOUSEHOLD MEASURE |
|------|------|------|
| Anchovette fish spread | ¾ oz | 1 tbsp |
| Apricot 100% Pure Fruit spread, no added sugar | ½ oz | 1 tbsp |
| Apricot fruit spread, reduced sugar | ½ oz | 1 tbsp |
| Butter | ⅓ oz | 2 tsp |
| Cashew spread | ⅓ oz | 2 tsp |
| Cottee's 100% Fruit Jam Apricot | 1 oz | 1 tbsp |
| Cottee's 100% Fruit Jam Blackberry | 1 oz | 1 tbsp |
| Cottee's 100% Fruit Jam Breakfast Marmalade | 1 oz | 1 tbsp |
| Cottee's 100% Fruit Jam Raspberry | 1 oz | 1 tbsp |
| Cottee's 100% Fruit Jam Strawberry | 1 oz | 1 tbsp |
| Dairy blend, with canola oil | ⅓ oz | 2 tsp |
| Extra virgin olive oil spread | ¼ oz | 1 tsp |
| Fructose, pure | ½ oz | 3 tsp |
| Ginger Marmalade, original | ¾ oz | 2 tsp |
| Glucose tablets or powder | ½ oz | 1 tbsp |
| Glucose Syrup | ¾ oz | 3 tsp |
| Golden syrup | ¾ oz | 3 tsp |
| Honey, Capilano, blended | ¾ oz | 3 tsp |
| Honey, general | ¾ oz | 3 tsp |

@ part of GI symbol program       ★ little or no carbs

| CALORIES | FAT (g) | SATURATED FAT (g) | CARBO-HYDRATE (g) | FIBER (g) | SODIUM (mg) | GI | LOW MED HIGH |
|---|---|---|---|---|---|---|---|
| 4 | 2 | 1 | 1 | 0 | 240 | ★ | |
| 38 | 0 | 0 | 9 | 0 | 2 | 43 | low |
| 20 | 0 | 0 | 6 | 0 | 10 | 55 | low |
| 0 | 9 | 6 | 0 | 0 | 78 | ★ | |
| 2 | 5 | 1 | 3 | 1 | 2 | ★ | |
| 64 | 0 | 0 | 15 | 0 | 3 | 50 | low |
| 66 | 0 | 0 | 15 | 0 | 3 | 46 | low |
| 68 | 0 | 0 | 17 | 0 | 3 | 55 | low |
| 66 | 0 | 0 | 15 | 0 | 3 | 46 | low |
| 65 | 0 | 0 | 15 | 0 | 3 | 46 | low |
| 0 | 8 | 4 | 0 | 0 | 52 | ★ | |
| 0 | 4 | 1 | 0 | 0 | 18 | ★ | |
| 61 | 0 | 0 | 15 | 0 | 0 | 19 | low |
| 56 | 0 | 0 | 14 | 0 | 2 | 50 | low |
| 59 | 0 | 0 | 15 | 0 | 2 | 100 | high |
| 65 | 0 | 0 | 16 | 0 | 29 | 100 | high |
| 58 | 0 | 0 | 15 | 0 | 26 | 63 | med |
| 70 | 0 | 0 | 18 | 0 | 3 | 64 | med |
| 70 | 0 | 0 | 18 | 0 | 3 | 52 | low |

# SPREADS & SWEETENERS

| FOOD | SERVING SIZE | HOUSEHOLD MEASURE |
|------|------|------|
| Honey, Ironbark | ¾ oz | 3 tsp |
| Honey, Red Gum | ¾ oz | 3 tsp |
| Honey, Salvation Jane | ¾ oz | 3 tsp |
| Honey, Stringybark | ¾ oz | 3 tsp |
| Honey, Yapunya | ¾ oz | 3 tsp |
| Honey, Yellow-box | ¾ oz | 3 tsp |
| Hummus (chickpea dip) | 1 oz | 1½ tbsp |
| Jam, sweetened with aspartame | ⅓ oz | 2 tsp |
| Jam, sweetened with sucralose | ⅓ oz | 2 tsp |
| Jelly, grape | ½ oz | 1 packet |
| Lemon butter, homemade | ⅓ oz | 2 tsp |
| Maple flavored syrup, Cottee's® | ¾ oz | 3 tsp |
| Maple syrup, pure, Canadian | ¾ oz | 3 tsp |
| Margarine, canola | ⅓ oz | 2 tsp |
| Marmalade, orange | ½ oz | 1 tbsp |
| Marmalade, sweetened with aspartame | ⅓ oz | 2 tsp |
| Marmalade, sweetened with sucralose | ⅓ oz | 2 tsp |
| Nutella®, hazelnut spread | 1 oz | 1½ tbsp |
| @ Premium Agave Nectar, Sweet Cactus Farms | ¾ oz | 4 tsp |
| President's Choice® Blue Menu™ Twice the Fruit Apricot spread | ½ oz | 1 tbsp |

@ part of GI symbol program     ★ little or no carbs

| CALORIES | FAT (g) | SATURATED FAT (g) | CARBO-HYDRATE (g) | FIBER (g) | SODIUM (mg) | GI | LOW MED HIGH |
|---|---|---|---|---|---|---|---|
| 70 | 0 | 0 | 18 | 0 | 3 | 48 | low |
| 70 | 0 | 0 | 18 | 0 | 3 | 53 | low |
| 70 | 0 | 0 | 18 | 0 | 3 | 64 | med |
| 70 | 0 | 0 | 18 | 0 | 3 | 44 | low |
| 0 | 0 | 0 | 18 | 0 | 3 | 52 | low |
| 0 | 0 | 0 | 18 | 0 | 3 | 35 | low |
| 73 | 5 | 1 | 6 | 3 | 93 | 22 | low |
| 0 | 0 | 0 | 0 | 0 | 8 | ★ | |
| 0 | 0 | 0 | 0 | 0 | 8 | ★ | |
| 42 | 0 | 0 | 10 | 0 | 5 | 52 | low |
| 1 | 2 | 1 | 3 | 0 | 18 | ★ | |
| 58 | 0 | 0 | 15 | 0 | 10 | 68 | med |
| 52 | 0 | 0 | 13 | 0 | 2 | 54 | low |
| 0 | 7 | 1 | 0 | 0 | 79 | ★ | |
| 37 | 0 | 0 | 13 | 0 | 11 | 48 | low |
| 0 | 0 | 0 | 0 | 0 | 3 | ★ | |
| 0 | 0 | 0 | 0 | 0 | 3 | ★ | |
| 157 | 10 | 3 | 17 | 0 | 15 | 33 | low |
| 64 | 0 | 0 | 16 | 0 | 3 | 19 | low |
| 25 | 0 | 0 | 6 | 0 | 2 | 49 | low |

# SPREADS & SWEETENERS

| FOOD | SERVING SIZE | HOUSEHOLD MEASURE |
|------|------|------|
| President's Choice® Blue Menu™ Twice the Fruit Spread— Strawberry & Rhubarb | ½ oz | 1 tbsp |
| Raspberry 100% Pure Fruit spread, no added sugar | ½ oz | 1 tbsp |
| Strawberry jam, regular | ¾ oz | 3 tsp |
| Sugar, brown | ½ oz | 6 tsp |
| Sugar, white | ½ oz | 6 tsp |
| @ Sweetaddin | ½ oz | 3 tsp |
| Tahini | ¾ oz | 1 tbsp |
| Treacle | ¾ oz | 3 tsp |

| CALORIES | FAT (g) | SATURATED FAT (g) | CARBO-HYDRATE (g) | FIBER (g) | SODIUM (mg) | GI | LOW MED HIGH |
|---|---|---|---|---|---|---|---|
| 25 | 0 | 0 | 6 | 0 | 0 | 69 | med |
| 39 | 0 | 0 | 9 | 0 | 2 | 26 | low |
| 53 | 0 | 0 | 13 | 0 | 3 | 51 | low |
| 65 | 0 | 0 | 17 | 0 | 2 | 61 | med |
| 65 | 0 | 0 | 17 | 0 | 2 | 65 | med |
| 61 | 0 | 0 | 15 | 0 | 0 | 19 | low |
| 4 | 12 | 2 | 0 | 0 | 16 | ★ | |
| 51 | 0 | 0 | 13 | 0 | 36 | 68 | med |

## Nutritive Sweeteners

### Fructose

| | |
|---|---|
| GI 19<br>4 cal (16 kJ) per gram<br>11 cal (46 kJ) per teaspoon table sugar equivalent* | Fructose or fruit sugar has a relatively small effect on blood glucose levels. It is sweeter than table sugar, but has the same number of calories per gram.<br><br>Sweetness relative to table sugar = up to 70% more, depending on the temperature of the food |

### Glucose

| | |
|---|---|
| GI 100<br>4 cal (16 kJ) per gram<br>26 cal (108 kJ) per teaspoon table sugar equivalent* | Glucose is the sugar found in blood. When eaten, it causes blood glucose levels to rise rapidly. It is not as sweet as table sugar, but has the same number of calories per gram.<br><br>Sweetness relative to table sugar = 25% less |

### Golden syrup

| | |
|---|---|
| GI 63<br>3 cal (12 kJ) per gram<br>11 cal (45 kJ) per teaspoon table sugar equivalent* | Golden syrup has a moderate effect on blood glucose levels, very similar to table sugar. It is sweeter than table sugar, and has fewer calories per gram.<br><br>Sweetness relative to table sugar = 33% more |

* The number of calories in the volume of alternative sweetener that provides the equivalent sweetness to 1 teaspoon of table sugar.

## Nutritive Sweeteners

### Grape syrup

GI 52

4 cal (16 kJ) per gram

16 cal (68 kJ) per teaspoon table sugar equivalent*

Grape syrup or nectar has a moderate effect on blood glucose levels. It is a little sweeter than table sugar, but has the same number of calories.

Sweetness relative to table sugar = 20% more

### Honey

GI 35–64

4 cal (16 kJ) per gram

20 cal (83 kJ) per teaspoon table sugar equivalent*

Honey has a variable effect on blood glucose levels depending on whether it is a blend or a pure floral honey. The pure floral honeys appear to have lower GIs. On average, honey is slightly less sweet than table sugar, but has about the same number of calories per teaspoon.

Sweetness relative to table sugar = about the same

### Isomalt

GI 60

3 cal (11 kJ) per gram

26 cal (110 kJ) per teaspoon table sugar equivalent*

Isomalt has a moderate effect on blood glucose levels similar to table sugar. It is only half as sweet as table sugar, but has fewer calories, and may have a laxative effect if eaten in large quantities.

Sweetness relative to table sugar = half as sweet

# Nutritive Sweeteners

## Lactose

GI 46

4 cal (16 kJ) per gram

120 cal (500 kJ) per teaspoon table sugar equivalent*

Lactose is the sugar found in milk. It causes blood glucose levels to rise slowly. It is not very sweet at all, but has the same number of calories as table sugar.

Sweetness relative to table sugar = 85% less sweet

## Maltitol

GI 69

3 cal (13 kJ) per gram

21 cal (87 kJ) per teaspoon table sugar equivalent*

Maltitol has a moderate to high effect on blood glucose levels greater than that of table sugar. It is only three-quarters as sweet as table sugar, and has the same number of calories, and may have a laxative effect and cause flatulence and diarrhea if eaten in large quantities.

Sweetness relative to table sugar = 25% less sweet

## Maltodextrin

GI not known

4 cal (16 kJ) per gram

35 cal (146 kJ) per teaspoon table sugar equivalent*

The effect of maltodextrin on blood glucose levels is not exactly known, though it is likely to be similar to that of glucose. It is only half as sweet as table sugar, and has the same number of calories. Sweetness relative to table sugar = half as sweet

---

\* The number of calories in the volume of alternative sweetener that provides the equivalent sweetness to 1 teaspoon of table sugar.

## Nutritive Sweeteners

### Maltose

GI 105

4 cal (16 kJ) per gram

60 cal (250 kJ) per teaspoon table sugar equivalent*

Maltose or malt causes blood glucose levels to rise rapidly. It is only one-third as sweet as table sugar, and has the same number of calories.

Sweetness relative to table sugar = 67% less sweet

### Mannitol

GI n/a

2 cal (9 kJ) per gram

15 cal (64 kJ) per teaspoon table sugar equivalent*

Mannitol has essentially no effect on blood glucose levels. It is only three-quarters as sweet as table sugar, but has only half the amount of calories, and may have a laxative effect and cause gas and diarrhea if eaten in large quantities.

Sweetness relative to table sugar = 25% less sweet

### Maple syrup

GI 54

3 cal (11 kJ) per gram

15 cal (61 kJ) per teaspoon table sugar equivalent*

Real maple syrup has a moderate effect on blood glucose levels. It is a little sweeter than table sugar, but has fewer calories. Sweetness relative to table sugar = 10% more

# Nutritive Sweeteners

## Polydextrose

GI 7

1 cal (5 kJ) per gram

6 cal (25 kJ) per teaspoon table sugar equivalent*

Polydextrose has very little effect on blood glucose levels. It is not sweet, but is used as a bulking agent with nonnutritive sweeteners. It has only one-third the amount of calories as table sugar, but may have a laxative effect if eaten in large quantities.

Sweetness relative to table sugar = not sweet

## Table sugar (sucrose)

GI 60 (average)

4 cal (16 kJ) per gram

16 cal (67 kJ) per teaspoon

Sucrose or table sugar is the most common sweetener eaten in North America. Despite popular misconceptions, it causes blood glucose levels to rise only moderately (less than white bread).

Sweetness = 100%
Castor sugar, brown sugar, raw sugar, confectioners' sugar are all forms of sugar.

## Xylitol

GI 21

3 cal (12 kJ) per gram

14 cal (60 kJ) per teaspoon table sugar equivalent*

Xylitol is a sugar alcohol that has little effect on blood glucose levels. It is as sweet as sugar and has fewer calories, but may have a laxative effect and cause gas and diarrhea if consumed in large quantities. Sweetness relative to table sugar = 100% as sweet

* The number of calories in the volume of alternative sweetener that provides the equivalent sweetness to 1 teaspoon of table sugar.

# Nonnutritive Sweeteners

## Acesulphame potassium or Acesulphame K

GI 0

0 cal (0 kJ) per gram

0 cal (0 kJ) per teaspoon table sugar equivalent*

Food additive code 950

Brand names: Sweet One, Sunett

Acesulphame K is much sweeter than sugar, has no effect on blood glucose levels, and doesn't provide any calories because it is not absorbed into the body.

Sweetness relative to table sugar = 200 times more

## Aspartame

GI 0

4 cal (17 kJ) per gram

0.3 cal (1.4 kJ) per teaspoon table sugar equivalent*

Brand names: Nutrasweet, Equal, Equal Spoonful

Aspartame is a couple of hundred times sweeter than sugar, and has essentially no effect on blood glucose levels. Because it is a protein it does provide some calories, but because it is very sweet, you only use it in small amounts.

Sweetness relative to table sugar = 150–250 times more

Warning: Aspartame should not be used by people with phenylketonuria.

## Nonnutritive Sweeteners

### Neotame

GI 0

4 cal (17 kJ) per gram

0 cal (0 kJ) per teaspoon table sugar equivalent*

Neotame is many thousands of times sweeter than sugar, and has essentially no effect on blood glucose levels. Because it is a protein it does provide some calories, but because it is extremely sweet, it is only used in tiny amounts.

Sweetness relative to table sugar = 7,000–13,000 times more

While neotame is approved by the Food and Drug Administration (FDA), it is not currently found in many foods or beverages.

### Saccharin

GI 0

0 cal (0 kJ) per gram

0 cal (0 kJ) per teaspoon table sugar equivalent*

Brand names: Sweet 'n Low, Sugar Twin

Saccharin is hundreds of times sweeter than sugar, has no effect on blood glucose levels, and is not metabolized by the human body.

Sweetness relative to table sugar = 300–500 times mo

### Stevia

GI 0

2.7 cal (11 kJ) per gram

0.7 cal (3 kJ) per teaspoon table sugar equivalent*

Stevia is considerably sweeter than sugar and has essentially no effect on blood glucose levels.

Sweetness relative to table sugar = 30 times more

---

* The number of calories in the volume of alternative sweetener that provides the equivalent sweetness to 1 teaspoon of table sugar.

## Nonnutritive Sweeteners

### Sucralose

GI 0

0 cal (0 kJ) per gram

0 cal (0 kJ) per teaspoon
table sugar equivalent*

Brand name: Splenda

Sucralose is hundreds of times sweeter than sugar, has no effect on blood glucose levels, and does not provide any calories because it is not absorbed into the body.

Sweetness relative to table sugar = 400–600 times more

# VEGETABLES

| FOOD | SERVING SIZE | HOUSEHOLD MEASURE |
|---|---|---|
| Alfalfa sprouts | ½ oz | 6 tbsp |
| Artichoke, globe | 4 oz | 1 medium |
| Artichoke hearts, whole, canned | 1½ oz | 1 heart |
| Artichokes in brine | 1½ oz | 1 heart |
| Artichoke hearts in brine, drained | 3 oz | 2 hearts |
| Arugula | ¾ oz | 3 medium leaves |
| Asparagus | 3 oz | 8 small spears |
| Asparagus, canned, drained | 3 oz | ¾ cup |
| Asparagus green/white spears, canned | 2 oz | ½ cup |
| Asparagus in springwater | 2 oz | ½ cup |
| Baby corn, cut, canned | 1¾ oz | ⅓ cup |
| Baby corn spears, whole, canned | 1¾ oz | ⅓ cup |
| Bamboo shoots, canned | 1 oz | ¼ cup |
| Bean sprouts, cooked | 2 oz | ½ cup |
| Bean sprouts, raw | 1 oz | ⅓ cup |
| Beans, green | 1¾ oz | 10 beans |
| Beans, Chinese long | 2½ oz | ½ cup |
| Beets, canned | 6 oz | 1 cup sliced |
| Bok choy | 3 oz | ½ cup |
| Broccoflower | 1½ oz | ½ cup |
| Broccoli | 3½ oz | 1 cup |
| Brussels sprouts | 2¾ oz | 4 sprouts |
| Cabbage, Chinese | 3 oz | ½ cup |

@ part of GI symbol program   ★ little or no carbs

| CALORIES | FAT (g) | SATURATED FAT (g) | CARBO-HYDRATE (g) | FIBER (g) | SODIUM (mg) | GI | LOW MED HIGH |
|---|---|---|---|---|---|---|---|
| 4 | 0 | 0 | 0 | 0 | 7 | ★ | |
| 28 | 0 | 0 | 2 | 1 | 7 | ★ | |
| 14 | 0 | 0 | 1 | 0 | 80 | ★ | |
| 12 | 0 | 0 | 2 | 0 | 130 | ★ | |
| 19 | 0 | 0 | 1 | 2 | 249 | ★ | |
| 6 | 0 | 0 | 1 | 0 | 6 | ★ | |
| 20 | 0 | 0 | 1 | 1 | 2 | ★ | |
| 22 | 0 | 0 | 1 | 4 | 216 | ★ | |
| 12 | 0 | 0 | 1 | 0 | 104 | ★ | |
| 8 | 0 | 0 | 1 | 0 | 110 | ★ | |
| 13 | 0 | 0 | 2 | 1 | 135 | ★ | |
| 13 | 0 | 0 | 2 | 1 | 105 | ★ | |
| 4 | 0 | 0 | 0 | 1 | 3 | ★ | |
| 16 | 0 | 0 | 1 | 2 | 1 | ★ | |
| 6 | 0 | 0 | 0 | 0 | 69 | ★ | |
| 14 | 0 | 0 | 1 | 2 | 2 | ★ | |
| 21 | 0 | 0 | 1 | 3 | 1 | ★ | |
| 82 | 0 | 0 | 16 | 5 | 540 | 64 | med |
| 30 | 2 | 1 | 1 | 1 | 21 | ★ | |
| 13 | 0 | 0 | 1 | 1 | 8 | ★ | |
| 34 | 0 | 0 | 1 | 4 | 20 | ★ | |
| 25 | 0 | 0 | 2 | 3 | 23 | ★ | |
| 29 | 2 | 1 | 1 | 1 | 18 | ★ | |

# VEGETABLES

| FOOD | SERVING SIZE | HOUSEHOLD MEASURE |
|------|------|------|
| Cabbage, green, cooked | 3 oz | ½ cup |
| Cabbage, green, raw | 3 oz | 1 cup |
| Cabbage, red, cooked | 3 oz | ½ cup |
| Cabbage, red, raw | 3 oz | 1 cup |
| Carrots, peeled, boiled | 3 oz | ½ cup |
| Cauliflower | 3 oz | ¾ cup |
| Celery, cooked | 2½ oz | 2 medium stalks |
| Celery, raw | 1 oz | 2 small stalks |
| Chili, banana, cooked | 1¾ oz | 1 average |
| Chili, banana, raw | 2 oz | 1 average |
| Chili, hot thin, cooked | ¾ oz | 1 average |
| Chili, hot thin, raw | 1 oz | 1 average |
| Chives | ¼ oz | 1 tbsp |
| Chayote | 1½ oz | ¼ average |
| Cucumber | 1 oz | 3 slices |
| Cucumber, Persian | 1 oz | 3 slices |
| Eggplant, cooked | 1¾ oz | 1 slice |
| Eggplant, raw | 1½ oz | ½ cup |
| Endive | 3 oz | ½ cup |
| Fennel, cooked | 2½ oz | ½ cup |
| Fennel, raw | 1¾ oz | ½ cup |
| Garlic | ¼ oz | 1 clove |
| Ginger | ⅒ oz | 1 tsp |

@ part of GI symbol program    ★ little or no carbs

| CALORIES | FAT (g) | SATURATED FAT (g) | CARBO-HYDRATE (g) | FIBER (g) | SODIUM (mg) | GI | LOW MED HIGH |
|---|---|---|---|---|---|---|---|
| 20 | 0 | 0 | 2 | 3 | 15 | ★ | |
| 23 | 0 | 0 | 2 | 3 | 17 | ★ | |
| 26 | 0 | 0 | 3 | 3 | 14 | ★ | |
| 30 | 0 | 0 | 3 | 4 | 15 | ★ | |
| 30 | 0 | 0 | 6 | 2 | 49 | 39 | low |
| 21 | 0 | 0 | 2 | 2 | 13 | ★ | |
| 13 | 0 | 0 | 2 | 2 | 63 | ★ | |
| 5 | 0 | 0 | 1 | 1 | 28 | ★ | |
| 10 | 0 | 0 | 1 | 1 | 2 | ★ | |
| 10 | 0 | 0 | 1 | 1 | 2 | ★ | |
| 6 | 0 | 0 | 1 | 1 | 1 | ★ | |
| 9 | 0 | 0 | 1 | 1 | 1 | ★ | |
| 1 | 0 | 0 | 0 | 0 | 0 | ★ | |
| 9 | 0 | 0 | 2 | 1 | 3 | ★ | |
| 3 | 0 | 0 | 0 | 0 | 5 | ★ | |
| 4 | 0 | 0 | 1 | 0 | 5 | ★ | |
| 12 | 0 | 0 | 1 | 1 | 2 | ★ | |
| 9 | 0 | 0 | 1 | 1 | 2 | ★ | |
| 16 | 0 | 0 | 0 | 2 | 81 | ★ | |
| 20 | 0 | 0 | 3 | 3 | 26 | ★ | |
| 12 | 0 | 0 | 2 | 1 | 19 | ★ | |
| 4 | 0 | 0 | 0 | 1 | 0 | ★ | |
| 0 | 0 | 0 | 0 | 0 | 0 | ★ | |

# VEGETABLES

| FOOD | SERVING SIZE | HOUSEHOLD MEASURE |
|------|------|------|
| Green beans, sliced, canned | 3 oz | ⅓ cup |
| Green plantain, peeled, boiled, 10 min | 4 oz | ½ cup |
| Green plantain, peeled, fried in vegetable oil | 4 oz | ½ cup |
| Hash browns | 2 oz | 1 average |
| Herbs, fresh or dried | ¹⁄₁₀ oz | 1 tsp |
| Horseradish | ¼ oz | 1 average |
| Kohlrabi | 3 oz | ½ cup |
| Leeks, cooked | 3 oz | 1 average |
| Leeks, raw | 3 oz | 1 average |
| Lettuce, cos | ¾ oz | 3 medium leaves |
| Lettuce, iceberg | ¾ oz | 3 medium leaves |
| Lettuce, mignonette | ¾ oz | 3 medium leaves |
| Mashed potato, made with milk | 4 oz | ½ cup |
| Mashed potato, made with milk and margarine | 4.2 oz | ½ cup |
| Mixed vegetables, Chinese, canned | 3 oz | ⅓ cup |
| Mushrooms | 1¼ oz | ½ cup |
| Mushrooms, canned | 1 oz | 3 small |
| Mushrooms, shiitake, canned | 1 oz | 3 small |
| Okra | 3 oz | ½ cup |
| Onion | 1 oz | ½ medium |
| Onions, canned, sautéed and diced | 1¾ oz | 1 medium |

@ part of GI symbol program  ★ little or no carbs

| CALORIES | FAT (g) | SATURATED FAT (g) | CARBO-HYDRATE (g) | FIBER (g) | SODIUM (mg) | GI | LOW MED HIGH |
|---|---|---|---|---|---|---|---|
| 30 | 0 | 0 | 5 | 3 | 281 | ★ | |
| 150 | 1 | 0 | 37 | 3 | 5 | 39 | low |
| 194 | 6 | 1 | 37 | 3 | 5 | 40 | low |
| 171 | 12 | 5 | 15 | 1 | 281 | 75 | high |
| 0 | 0 | 0 | 0 | 0 | 0 | ★ | |
| 4 | 0 | 0 | 1 | 0 | 0 | ★ | |
| 36 | 0 | 0 | 4 | 3 | 12 | ★ | |
| 27 | 0 | 0 | 3 | 2 | 13 | ★ | |
| 28 | 0 | 0 | 3 | 3 | 14 | ★ | |
| 5 | 0 | 0 | 0 | 1 | 4 | ★ | |
| 2 | 0 | 0 | 0 | 0 | 5 | ★ | |
| 4 | 0 | 0 | 0 | 1 | 4 | ★ | |
| 82 | 1 | 0 | 15 | 2 | 10 | 85 | high |
| 117 | 4 | 1 | 20 | 2 | 350 | 71 | high |
| 26 | 0 | 0 | 5 | 1 | 68 | ★ | |
| 11 | 0 | 0 | 1 | 1 | 3 | ★ | |
| 11 | 1 | 0 | 1 | 1 | 5 | ★ | |
| 8 | 0 | 0 | 1 | 1 | 96 | ★ | |
| 29 | 0 | 0 | 1 | 4 | 2 | ★ | |
| 13 | 0 | 0 | 2 | 1 | 4 | ★ | |
| 26 | 1 | 0 | 3 | 1 | 215 | ★ | |

# VEGETABLES

| FOOD | SERVING SIZE | HOUSEHOLD MEASURE |
|---|---|---|
| Onions, sautèed and diced | ½ oz | I medium slice |
| Parsley, cooked | 1 ½ oz | ½ cup |
| Parsley, raw | ¼ oz | I tbsp |
| Parsnips, boiled | 2¾ oz | ½ cup |
| Peas, green | 7 oz | 1½ cups |
| Pepper, green, canned | 1½ oz | ¼ cup |
| Pepper, green, raw | 1½ oz | 4 rings |
| Pepper, red, canned | 1½ oz | ¼ cup |
| Pepper, red, cooked | 1½ oz | 4 rings |
| Potato, baked, without skin | 3½ oz | I medium |
| Potato chips, deep fried | 1½ oz | 10 average chips |
| Potatoes, Baked, Russet Burbank potatoes, baked, without fat | 5.75 oz | I med potato |
| Potatoes, boiled | 5.75 oz | I med potato |
| Potatoes, Désirée, peeled, boiled 35 mins | 4 oz | I medium (2¾-inch diameter) |
| Potato, instant, mashed, Idahoan | 4 oz | ½ cup, prepared |
| Potatoes, Nardine, peeled, boiled | 4 oz | I medium (2¾-inch diameter) |
| Potatoes, new, canned, microwaved 3 mins | 5 oz | 4 small (1-inch diameter) |
| Potatoes, new, unpeeled, boiled 20 mins | 5 oz | 4 small (1-inch diameter) |

@ part of GI symbol program   ★ little or no carbs

| CALORIES | FAT (g) | SATURATED FAT (g) | CARBO-HYDRATE (g) | FIBER (g) | SODIUM (mg) | GI | LOW MED HIGH |
|---|---|---|---|---|---|---|---|
| 6 | 0 | 0 | 1 | 0 | 2 | ★ | |
| 10 | 0 | 0 | 0 | 2 | 21 | ★ | |
| 1 | 0 | 0 | 0 | 0 | 2 | ★ | |
| 16 | 0 | 0 | 8 | 1 | 1 | 52 | low |
| 128 | 0 | 0 | 15 | 13 | 2 | 45 | low |
| 8 | 0 | 0 | 1 | 0 | 1 | ★ | |
| 7 | 0 | 0 | 1 | 0 | 1 | ★ | |
| 12 | 0 | 0 | 2 | 1 | 0 | ★ | |
| 11 | 0 | 0 | 2 | 1 | 0 | ★ | |
| 72 | 0 | 0 | 14 | 1 | 8 | 85 | high |
| 126 | 7 | 3 | 14 | 1 | 72 | 75 | high |
| 168 | 0 | 0 | 41 | 4 | 24 | 76 | high |
| 144 | 0 | 0 | 36 | 3 | 8 | 59 | med |
| 82 | 0 | 0 | 16 | 2 | 4 | 101 | high |
| 170 | 0 | 0 | 16 | 2 | 15 | 88 | high |
| 82 | 0 | 0 | 16 | 2 | 4 | 70 | high |
| 84 | 0 | 0 | 16 | 2 | 470 | 65 | med |
| 84 | 0 | 0 | 16 | 2 | 4 | 78 | high |

# VEGETABLES

| FOOD | SERVING SIZE | HOUSEHOLD MEASURE |
|---|---|---|
| Potatoes, Ontario, white, baked in skin | 5.75 oz | I med potato |
| Potatoes, Pontiac, peeled, boiled 15 mins, mashed | 4 oz | ½ cup |
| Potatoes, Pontiac, peeled, boiled whole 30–35 mins | 4 oz | I medium (2¾ inch diameter) |
| Potatoes, Pontiac, peeled, microwaved 7 mins | 4 oz | I medium (2¾ inch diameter) |
| Potatoes, red, boiled with skin on in salted water 12 min | 5.75 oz | I med potato |
| Potato, red, cubed, boiled in salted water 12 min, stored overnight in refrigerator, consumed cold | 5.75 oz | I med potato |
| Potatoes, Sebago, peeled, boiled 35 mins | 4 oz | I medium (2¾ inch diameter) |
| Potato, wedge, with skin | I¼ oz | 2 small |
| Potato salad, canned | 4 oz | ½ cup |
| Pumpkin, boiled | 7½ oz | I¼ cup |
| Radishes, red | 2 oz | 6 large |
| Rutabaga | 5.75 oz | I cup sliced |
| Sauerkraut, canned | 2½ oz | ½ cup |
| Seaweed | I½ oz | ½ cup |
| Shallots, cooked | I oz | 3 medium |
| Shallots, raw | ½ oz | 2 average |
| Snowpeas, cooked | 2¾ oz | 20 average |
| Snowpeas, raw | I oz | 10 average |

@ part of GI symbol program     ★ little or no carbs

| CALORIES | FAT (g) | SATURATED FAT (g) | CARBO-HYDRATE (g) | FIBER (g) | SODIUM (mg) | GI | LOW MED HIGH |
|---|---|---|---|---|---|---|---|
| 161 | 0 | 0 | 41 | 4 | 17 | 60 | med |
| 74 | 0 | 0 | 14 | 2 | 4 | 91 | high |
| 82 | 0 | 0 | 16 | 2 | 4 | 72 | high |
| 82 | 0 | 0 | 16 | 2 | 4 | 79 | high |
| 148 | 0 | 0 | 37 | 3 | 7 | 89 | high |
| 148 | 0 | 0 | 37 | 3 | 7 | 56 | med |
| 82 | 0 | 0 | 16 | 2 | 4 | 87 | high |
| 118 | 4 | 1 | 17 | 2 | 23 | 75 | high |
| 147 | 8 | 2 | 16 | 1 | 408 | 63 | med |
| 96 | 1 | 1 | 15 | 3 | 2 | 66 | med |
| 9 | 0 | 0 | 1 | 1 | 12 | ★ | |
| 66 | 0 | 0 | 18 | 3 | 34 | 72 | high |
| 12 | 0 | 0 | 1 | 3 | 322 | ★ | |
| 13 | 0 | 0 | 0 | 5 | 60 | ★ | |
| 9 | 0 | 0 | 1 | 0 | 33 | ★ | |
| 4 | 0 | 0 | 1 | 0 | 16 | ★ | |
| 39 | 0 | 0 | 4 | 2 | 1 | ★ | |
| 12 | 0 | 0 | 2 | 1 | 0 | ★ | |

# VEGETABLES

| FOOD | SERVING SIZE | HOUSEHOLD MEASURE |
|---|---|---|
| Spinach, cooked | 3 oz | ⅔ cup |
| Spinach, raw | 1 oz | 1 cup |
| Spring onions | ½ oz | 1 medium |
| Squash | 2½ oz | 2 average |
| Squash, butternut, boiled | 2¾ oz | ½ cup |
| Sweet corn, Honey 'n Pearl variety, boiled | 2¾ oz | 1 medium (5 inches long) |
| Sweet corn, on the cob, boiled | 2¾ oz | 1 medium (5 inches long) |
| Sweet corn, whole kernel, canned, drained | 3 oz | ½ cup |
| Sweet potato, baked | 3 oz | ½ large |
| Sweet potato, peeled, cubed, boiled in salted water 15 min | 5 oz | 1 med potato |
| Swiss chard | 4 oz | 1 cup |
| Taro, boiled | 1½ oz | ½ cup |
| Tomatoes | 1¾ oz | ½ small |
| Tomatoes, in tomato juice | 3 oz | ⅓ cup |
| Tomatoes, Italian diced | 4½ oz | ½ cup |
| Tomatoes, Italian whole peeled Roma | 4½ oz | ½ cup |
| Tomatoes, whole peeled, no added salt | 4½ oz | ½ cup |
| Tomato, onion, pepper, celery | 3 oz | ⅓ cup |
| Tomato puree | 2 oz | ¼ cup |

＠ part of GI symbol program   ★ little or no carbs

| CALORIES | FAT (g) | SATURATED FAT (g) | CARBO-HYDRATE (g) | FIBER (g) | SODIUM (mg) | GI | LOW MED HIGH |
|---|---|---|---|---|---|---|---|
| 28 | 0 | 0 | 1 | 6 | 18 | ★ | |
| 6 | 0 | 0 | 0 | 1 | 6 | ★ | |
| 5 | 0 | 0 | 1 | 0 | 0 | ★ | |
| 22 | 0 | 0 | 2 | 2 | 1 | ★ | |
| 30 | 0 | 0 | 6 | 2 | 2 | 51 | low |
| 84 | 1 | 0 | 15 | 2 | 6 | 37 | low |
| 84 | 1 | 0 | 15 | 2 | 6 | 48 | low |
| 90 | 1 | 0 | 16 | 3 | 238 | 46 | low |
| 79 | 0 | 0 | 16 | 2 | 12 | 46 | low |
| 115 | 0 | 0 | 31 | 4 | 41 | 59 | med |
| 24 | 0 | 0 | 2 | 4 | 213 | ★ | |
| 63 | 0 | 0 | 15 | 2 | 7 | 54 | low |
| 9 | 0 | 0 | 1 | 1 | 3 | ★ | |
| 19 | 0 | 0 | 3 | 1 | 56 | ★ | |
| 28 | 1 | 1 | 5 | 2 | 125 | ★ | |
| 30 | 1 | 1 | 5 | 2 | 125 | ★ | |
| 25 | 0 | 0 | 4 | 1 | 6 | ★ | |
| 19 | 0 | 0 | 3 | 1 | 60 | ★ | |
| 20 | 0 | 0 | 3 | 1 | 221 | ★ | |

# VEGETABLES

| FOOD | SERVING SIZE | HOUSEHOLD* MEASURE |
|------|------|------|
| Turnips | 1¾ oz | ⅓ cup |
| Water chestnuts, drained | ¾ oz | 2 tbsp |
| Watercress | ¼ oz | ¼ cup |
| Yam, peeled, boiled | 2½ oz | ½ cup |
| Zucchini, cooked | 3 oz | 1 medium |
| Zucchini, raw | 2 oz | ½ medium |

| CALORIES | FAT (g) | SATURATED FAT (g) | CARBO-HYDRATE (g) | FIBER (g) | SODIUM (mg) | GI | LOW MED HIGH |
|---|---|---|---|---|---|---|---|
| 14 | 0 | 0 | 2 | 2 | 12 | ★ | |
| 11 | 0 | 0 | 2 | 1 | 2 | ★ | |
| 1 | 0 | 0 | 0 | 0 | 3 | ★ | |
| 79 | 0 | 0 | 16 | 3 | 5 | 54 | low |
| 17 | 0 | 0 | 2 | 2 | 1 | ★ | |
| 10 | 0 | 0 | 1 | 1 | 1 | ★ | |

# The online GI database

The glycemic index online search tool was developed in 2001 at the University of Sydney following the success of a similar database used to calculate the nutritional value of meals served at the Sydney Olympics in 2000. The tool, designed by Associate Professor Gareth Denyer, has proved to be very popular, with thousands of "hits" per week from all over the world. The GI database tool allows quick searches of the ever-growing number of foods tested over the past 25 years. The online tool reveals GI values, the glycemic load (GL), and grams of carbohydrate per serving on first glance. Dig a little deeper and you will see where and when the food was tested and also in whom the foods were tested (i.e., people with and without diabetes).

Some of our readers have written to us expressing difficulties in finding specific foods in the database. In the following paragraphs we illustrate the different features and tricks of searching the GI database and explain what the results mean.

1) First, click on the GI Database link in the left-hand menu at www.glycemicindex.com.

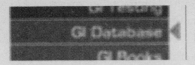

You will arrive at the main search page. To begin your search for a specific food, you will need to pay attention to the window shown below.

2) In this example, we will search for "beans." If beans are added into the Name field and the Search button is clicked (or just hit the Enter key on your keyboard), the result produces 96 different foods either containing beans or showing specific types of bean. To narrow down the results to something more manageable, why not use the other fields to refine your search? In the example shown below, we have also added information into the GI and GL field. By using the less than (<) and greater than (>) options, we can tell the database to show us only foods containing beans with a GI less than 55 and a GL less than 15.

3) Executing the search returns 69 foods fitting the
   search criteria. Let's say we are interested in refried
   beans. This first page shows us that refried pinto
   beans have a GI of 38, that one serving is 150 grams,
   that there are 26 grams of carbohydrate in the
   serving, and that the glycemic load (GL) is 10.

| Refried Pinto beans, Casa Fiesta™ brand (Capitol Foods Pty Ltd, Australia) | 38 | 150 | 26 | 10 |
|---|---|---|---|---|

## Database tips

1) Foods with no GI are not included in the database.
   If you search for olive oil, for example, there will
   be no result. Foods must contain an appreciable
   amount of available carbohydrate to have a GI
   value.

2) While the GI database is the most comprehensive
   resource on the web for GI and GL values, we
   have not tested every food in the world (some
   think we have!). In some cases certain companies
   choose to not reveal the GI of their products.
   In most cases they have not chosen to have a
   product tested at all. If you would like to see the
   GI value of a certain product, you might consider
   writing to the manufacturer and ask that it be
   tested.

3) For a quick list of the most recently tested foods,
   click on the "Last 6 or 12 Months" buttons below
   the main search fields.

4) Now click on the actual food name (the text will change color) and the following page appears.

---

Food Name and Manufacturer: **Refried Pinto Beans, Casa Fiesta™ brand (Capital Foods Pty Ltd, Australia)**

GI (vs Glucose): **3**

Serve Size: **150 grams**

Carb per Serve (g): **26**

Glycemic Load: **10**

Time Period of Test: **2 h**

Subjects Used in Test: **Normal**

Reference: **Sydney University's Glycemic Index Research Service (Human Nutrition Unit, University of Sydney, Australia) unpublished observations, 1995–2007.**

---

More detailed information on the specific food is displayed. The GI of these particular refried beans was calculated using glucose as the standard (i.e., glucose = 100). The +/- 3 refers to the standard error of the mean (SEM). Ideally, the SEM should be approximately 10% of the actual GI value. The serving (g) refers to the standard or nominal/usual serving size of that product—e.g., milk usually 1 glass (250–300 ml), pasta about 150 g, bread usually 2 slices (70 g), cereals usually 30 or 45 g. Foods that have "unusual" numbers refer to products that come prepackaged in that size (for example Pop Tarts = 36 g) or have an averaged standard serving (doughnut = 47 g). Even if the serving (g) refers to a prepackaged weight it still represents a usual or standard serving (Mars Bar serving = 60 g).

The carb/serving (g) is the amount of carbohydrate per standard serving. This value is then used to calculate the GL value for each product:

**Refried pinto beans**
Serving (g): 150 g
CHO/serving (g): 26
GI: 38
GL = 10

In this case the test period was the standard 2 hours where a total of 8 finger-prick blood samples were taken in 10 subjects over that period (this includes 2 fasting samples). The subjects were "normal," which means they were healthy volunteers. In some tests, "Type 2" refers to testing in people with type 2 diabetes. Finally, the reference shows where the food was tested and in which journal the results were published, if applicable.

# Where to go for further help

## For further information on GI

**www.glycemicindex.com**

This is the University of Sydney's glycemic index website where you can learn about GI and access the GI database, which includes the most up-to-date listing of the GI of foods that have been published in international scientific journals.

**www.gisymbol.com**

The Glycemic Index (GI) Symbol Program is a food labeling program with strict nutritional criteria that aims to help people make informed food choices. The site includes a complete listing of foods carrying the GI symbol.

**http://ginews.blogspot.com**

GI News is the University of Sydney Human Nutrition Unit's official glycemic index monthly newsletter. Subscribing is free.

For further information and advice, we recommend that you contact the following organizations.

## American Diabetes Association (ADA)

ADA is the nation's leading nonprofit health organization for people with diabetes in the United States, providing information on diabetes and diabetes prevention, as well as tips and resources for living well with diabetes. ADA

has offices nationwide; to find the office closest to you, call 800-DIABETES (800-342-2383).
www.diabetes.org

## American Heart Association

The American Heart Association has offices all around the country. Contact the Heartline at 800-AHA-USA-1 (800-242-8721) for information, or go to their website.
www.americanheart.org

## Canadian Diabetes Association

The Canadian Diabetes Association is the national peak consumer health organization for people with diabetes in Canada. The aim of the organization is to promote the health of Canadians through diabetes research, education, service, and advocacy.
800-BANTING (800-226-8464)
www.diabetes.ca

## Crisis Services Kids Helpline (United States)

877-KIDS-400 (877-543-1400)
www.kidscrisis.com

## Diabetes Educators

### In the United States

**American Association of Diabetes Educators (AADE)**
200 W. Madison St., Suite 800
Chicago, IL 60606
800-338-3633
www.aadenet.org

In Canada

**Canadian Diabetes Educator Certification Board**

2878 King Street

Caledon, ON L7C 0R3

905-838-4898

www.cdecb.ca

## Dietitians

In the United States

**American Dietetic Association**

120 South Riverside Plaza, Suite 2000

Chicago, Illinois 60606

800-877-1600

www.eatright.org

In Canada

**Dietitians of Canada**

480 University Avenue, Suite 604

Toronto, ON M5G 1V2

416-596-0857

www.dieticians.ca

## Exercise Specialists

**Personal Trainer's Network**

An international database for locating personal trainers.

www.personaltrainers.net

## In the United States
**American Physical Therapy Association**
800-999-APTA (800-999-2782)
www.apta.org and click on "Find a PT"

**American Society of Exercise Physiologists**
www.asep.org

## In Canada
**Canadian Physiotherapy Association**
800-387-8679
www.physiotherapy.ca and click on "Find a
Physiotherapist"

**Canadian Society for Exercise Physiology**
877-651-3755
www.csep.ca

# Gluten Intolerance and Celiac Disease
www.celiac.nih.gov
www.celiac.org
www.gluten.net
www.glutenfree.com

# Heart and Stroke Foundation (Canada)
Call 613-569-4361 to find the Heart and Stroke
Foundation office nearest you.
ww2.heartandstroke.ca

# HopeLine (United States)

800-394-HOPE (800-394-4673)

www.thehopeline.com

# Juvenile Diabetes Research Foundation International

800-533-CURE (800-533-2873)

www.jdrf.org and click on "Locations"

# Kids Help Phone (Canada)

800-668-6868

www.kidshelpphone.ca

# Mood Disorder Society of Canada

For anyone suffering from depression and all other mood disorders, including depression, bipolar disorders, and anxiety, Mood Disorder Society provides resources to find help.

519-824-5565

www.mooddisorderscanada.ca

# National Alliance on Mental Illness (NAMI) (United States)

NAMI provides information and support for people living with mental illnesses and their friends and family.

Info helpline: 800-950-NAMI (800-950-6264)

www.nami.org

## Podiatrists

### In the United States
**American Podiatric Medical Association**
www.apma.org

### In Canada
**Canadian Podiatric Medical Association**
www.podiatrycanada.org

## Quitline

If you need help to stop smoking, call
United States: 800-QUIT-NOW (800-784-8669)
Canada: 877-513-5333

# Acknowledgments

We would like to thank the dedicated GI testing team at SUGiRS—Karola Stockmann and Kai Lin Ek-Rhodes—and all our cheerful, well-fed, and patient volunteers. We would also like to thank Associate Professor Gareth Denyer for his invaluable help with the GI database and Dr. Alan Barclay from the GI Symbol program for the sugars and sweeteners information and for thoroughly checking the GI tables for us.

Thank you to dietitian Kate Marsh, who helped us with the Low GI gluten-free eating section, Philippa Sandall, and everyone at Hachette Livre Australia who has worked so hard on our behalf, especially Fiona Hazard, Vanessa Radnidge, Francesca Wardell, and Joan Beal.

# Also Available

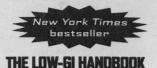
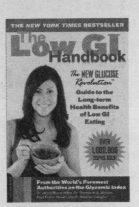

ISBN: 978-0-7382-1389-7
$16.95

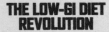

## THE LOW-GI HANDBOOK

Available in a new fourth edition in July 2010, the completely revised and updated *New York Times*-bestselling guide to the long-term benefits of low-GI eating.

## THE LOW-GI DIET REVOLUTION

The only science-based diet proven to help you lose up to 10 percent of your current weight and develop a lifetime of healthy eating habits.

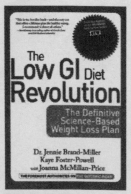

ISBN: 978-1-56924-413-5
$15.95

# THE NEW GLUCOSE REVOLUTION LIFE PLAN

With the glycemic index as its starting point, *The New Glucose Revolution Life Plan* gives readers clear guidelines for choosing the diet that is right for them.

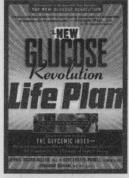

**ISBN: 978-1-56924-471-5**
**$18.95**

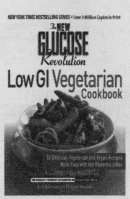

**ISBN-13: 978-1-56924-278-0**
**$19.95**

# THE NEW GLUCOSE REVOLUTION LOW GI VEGETARIAN COOKBOOK

The perfect cookbook for vegetarians and vegans looking to eat the right carbs. Features beautiful color photographs and more than 80 recipes low on the glycemic index.

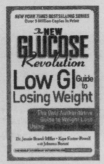

ISBN: 978-1-56924-336-7
$6.95

# THE NEW GLUCOSE REVOLUTION LOW GI GUIDE TO LOSING WEIGHT

*The New Glucose Revolution Low GI Guide to Losing Weight* describes the differences between carbohydrates and shows how eating low GI foods can help you burn body fat, foster good life-long eating habits, and maintain a healthy weight permanently.

# THE LOW GI DIET COOKBOOK

Features 100 easy-to-make, low-GI recipes–all of which feature low-GI carbohydrates–that will help you keep your weight under control and improve and maintain your overall health and vitality.

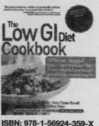

ISBN: 978-1-56924-359-X
$19.95

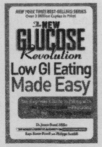

ISBN: 978-1-56924-385-5
$12.95

# THE NEW GLUCOSE REVOLUTION LOW GI EATING MADE EASY

This easy-to-follow guide features in-depth entries for the top 100 foods with the lowest GI values. Offers tips for making easy substitutions from high to low-GI foods and over 300 quick snacks, meals, and treats.